INFLUENZA - THERAPEUTICS AND CHALLENGES

Edited by **Shailendra K. Saxena**

Influenza - Therapeutics and Challenges
http://dx.doi.org/10.5772/intechopen.71939
Edited by Shailendra K. Saxena

Part of IntechOpen Book Series: Infectious Diseases, Volume 1
Book Series Editor: Shailendra K. Saxena

Contributors
Vsevolod Zinserling, Takuo Mizukami, Eita Sasaki, Isao Hamaguchi, Yulia A. Desheva, Clement Adebajo Meseko, Binod Kumar, Melvin Sanicas, Mikhail Kostinov, Ekaterina Khromova, Yuji Takemoto, Shailendra K. Saxena

First published in London, United Kingdom, 2018 by IntechOpen
IntechOpen is the global imprint of INTECHOPEN LIMITED, registered in England and Wales, registration number: 11086078, The Shard, 25th floor, 32 London Bridge Street
London, SE19SG – United Kingdom
Printed in Croatia

British Library Cataloguing-in-Publication Data
A catalogue record for this book is available from the British Library

Additional hard copies can be obtained from orders@intechopen.com

Influenza - Therapeutics and Challenges, Edited by Shailendra K. Saxena
p. cm.
Print ISBN 978-1-78923-714-6
Online ISBN 978-1-78923-715-3
ISSN 2631-6188

For EU product safety concerns:
IN TECH d.o.o., Prolaz Marije Krucifikse Kozulić 3, 51000 Rijeka, Croatia,
info@intechopen.com or visit our website at intechopen.com.

IntechOpen Book Series

Infectious Diseases

Volume 1

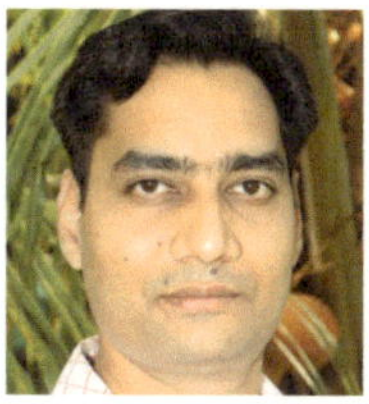

Prof. Shailendra K. Saxena is the vice dean and a professor at the Center for Advanced Research (CFAR), King George's Medical University (KGMU), Lucknow, in India. His research interests are to understand the molecular mechanisms of host defense during human viral infections and to develop new predictive, preventive, and therapeutic strategies for them using JEV, HIV, and oncogenic viruses as a model, via stem cells and cell culture technologies. His research work has been published in various high impact factor journals (Science, PNAS, Nature Medicine) with high citation. He has received many awards and honors in India and abroad including various Young Scientist Awards, BBSRC India Partnering Award, and Fellows and named as "Global Leader in Science" by The Scientist magazine (USA) and "International Opinion Leader/ Expert" involved in the vaccination for JE by IPIC (UK).

Book Series Editor: Shailendra K. Saxena
King George's Medical University

Scope of the Series

The series will give a most comprehensive overview of recent trends in various infectious diseases (as per the most recent Baltimore classification), as well as general concepts of infections, immunopathology, diagnosis, treatment, epidemiology and etiology to current clinical recommendations in management of infectious diseases, highlighting the ongoing issues, recent advances, with future directions in diagnostic approaches and therapeutic strategies. This book series will focus on various aspects and properties of infectious diseases whose deep understanding is very important for safeguarding human race from more loss of resources and economies due to pathogens.

Contents

Preface

Influenza is a perpetual economic burden causing significant morbidity and mortality rate in humans. Globally, the reported cases of seasonal influenza viruses rise up to 3–5 million during epidemics with estimated death toll of 290,000–650,000 per year. Comorbidity condition (such as diabetes and heart or liver disease) and immunocompromised condition of the patients are predominant causes of mortality associated with influenza virus. Transmission of influenza virus occurs by direct or indirect contact, inhaling virus-infected droplets or the small droplet nuclei, exposure to diseased poultry, intake of raw or undercooked poultry, or transplacental transmission. Influenza viruses enter humans through the respiratory tract by oral or nasal route, and then they cross the mucous layer surrounding the respiratory epithelium. The host defense mechanism gets activated to prohibit the spread of the virus. Innate and adaptive immune responses collectively play an important role in clearance of influenza virus from the host. A comprehensive understanding at the molecular and genetic level of the avian and swine influenza virus will strengthen us in understanding their mechanism of reassortment and transmission in humans. Several antivirals are given for the treatment of influenza virus infection such as adamantanes, oseltamivir, and zanamivir targeted toward viral proteins. The complementary and alternative medicine provides an additional support to the antivirals for its treatment. The development of the vaccine should consider several strategies such as epidemiological data of the previous pandemic influenza viruses, presence of viruses in nature, and viruses responsible for infecting human population. The current influenza vaccines available are live attenuated influenza vaccines (LAIV), inactivated influenza vaccine (IIV), recombinant subunit DNA, and vectored virus vaccine. There are some limitations associated with influenza virus vaccines suggesting circulating virus, and the vaccine virus should be of same strains to give a high efficacy, or else the vaccine might provide a false sense of security. Other preventive methods to control influenza are proper hand washing, the use of masks, covering the mouth during coughing and sneezing, avoiding physical contacts with influenza-infected individuals, wearing gloves while working with infected poultry or swine, and intake of effective antiviral medications. Awareness regarding the prevention and control methods of influenza should be widely spread.

This book covers a collection of articles by brilliant researchers who have devoted their time to combat influenza. This book gives a comprehensive overview of recent advances in influenza, as well as general concepts of molecular biology of influenza infections, epidemiology, immunopathology, prevention, and current clinical recommendations in management of influenza, including preparation of vaccines, assessment of the safety and quality of influenza vaccines and adjuvants highlighting the ongoing issues and recent advances, with future directions in prevention and therapeutic strategies. The book focuses on various aspects and properties of influenza, whose deep understanding is very important for safeguarding human race from more loss of resources and economies due to pathogens.

I hope that this work might increase the interest in this field of research and that the readers will find it useful for their investigations, management, and clinical usage. Also, I would like to thank our contributors, colleagues, family, and friends who gave us a lot of encouragement and support during the work on this book

Prof. Dr. Shailendra K. Saxena
FRSC (UK), FRSB (UK), FAcadTM (Austria), FBRS, FAEB,
FIVS, MNYAS (USA), MASM (USA), MASV (USA)
Center for Advanced Research
King George's Medical University (KGMU)
Lucknow, India

Section 1

Introduction

Chapter 1

Introductory Chapter: Human Influenza A Virus Infection - Global Prevalence, Prevention, Therapeutics, and Challenges

Shailendra K. Saxena, Amrita Haikerwal,
Swatantra Kumar and Madan L.B. Bhatt

Additional information is available at the end of the chapter

http://dx.doi.org/10.5772/intechopen.77350

1. Introduction

Influenza virus is a perpetual economic burden that causes a significant morbidity and mortality rate in humans. Globally, the reported cases of seasonal influenza viruses (SIVs) rise up to 3–5 million during epidemics with an estimated death toll of 290,000–650,000 per year [1]. The Global Influenza Surveillance and Response System (GISRS), a surveillance system of the World Health Organization (WHO), analyses the incidences of avian and zoonotic influenza virus to accurately estimate the severity of the disease. As of March 5–18, 2018, GISRS-WHO has reported 46.8% cases of influenza A virus (where 64% were influenza A(H1N1)pdm09 cases and 36% were infected with H3N2) and 53.2% of influenza B virus (where 91% were B-Yamagata strain and 9% were B-Victoria) [2]. The co-morbidity condition (such as diabetes, heart or liver disease) or the immuno-compromised condition of patients is the predominant cause of mortality associated with influenza virus.

Influenza virus belongs to the *Orthomyxoviridae* family and is categorized as influenza A virus (IAV), influenza B virus (IBV), and influenza C virus (ICV). The genome of influenza virus is segmented with 8 negative-sense single-stranded viral RNA (vRNA) strands which code for 11 proteins in cases of IAV and IAB, whereas IAC has seven vRNA segments that code for nine proteins. These segments are named after their main proteins such as segment 1-PB2 (polymerase basic 2), segment 2-PB1 (polymerase basic 1), segment 3-PA (polymerase acid), segment 4-HA (hemagglutinin), segment 5-NP (nucleoprotein), segment 6-NA (neuraminidase), segment 7-M (matrix), and segment 8-NS (non-structural) [3]. Influenza vRNA has heterotrimeric RNA-dependent RNA polymerase (RdRp) at the 5′ and 3′ end of the segment and the internal part of vRNA is bound with several nucleoproteins (NP) forming viral ribonucleoprotein complexes (vRNP) [4]. Hemagglutinin (HA) and neuraminidase (NA) are envelope glycoproteins responsible for the antigenic variation and the generation of different strains of influenza virus. HAs are of 16 subtypes (H1–H16) and NA has nine subtypes (N1-N9) [5]. As a result of the antigenic drift, SIVs are generated due to several point mutations in the *HA* and *NA* genes caused by RdRp [6]. Thus, the antibodies generated during primary infection with the influenza virus are unable to neutralize the drifted strains of SIVs, leading to epidemics or pandemics. Considerable numbers of individuals are always at risk of getting infected with influenza viruses, thus creating a state of alertness. In addition to SIVs, there are several pandemic viruses generated due to the antigenic shift, where the newly drifted strains of viruses have the ability to cross species barriers, as a result of the re-assortment of a viral genome with other influenza viruses (human or non-human).

2. Transmission

The natural reservoirs of IAV are duck and waterfowl allowing direct virus transmission to other avian hosts as well as in others via crossing species barrier such as in humans,

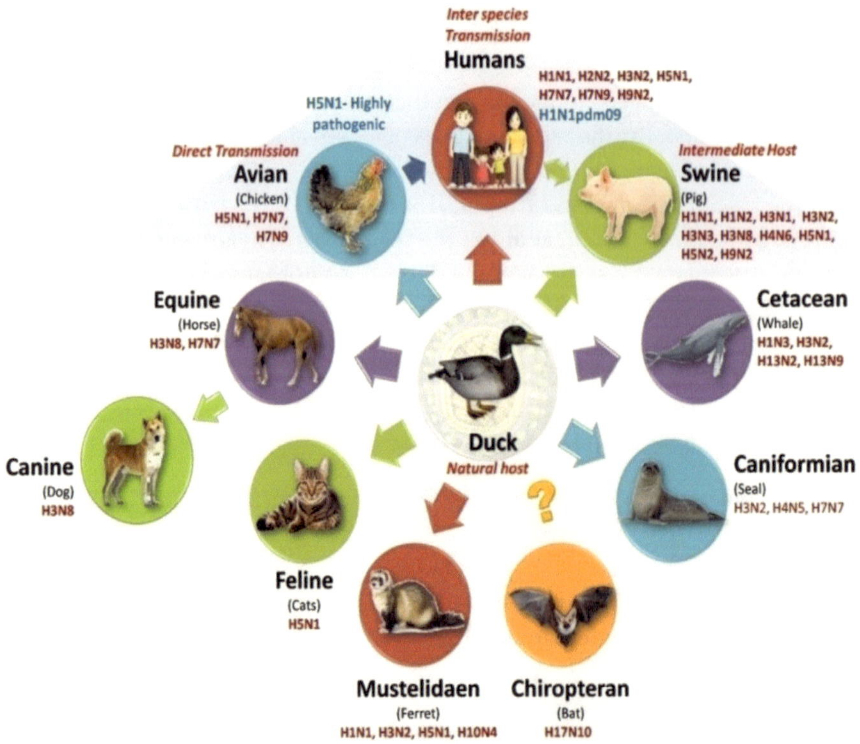

Figure 1. Transmission cycle of IAV: The triangle in the figure describes the most important transmission cycle of IAV, where the virus is directly transmitted from the natural host, duck to avian, and further transmitted to the human, or the virus is transmitted from duck to human by inter-species transmission or via pig where pig acts as an intermediate host between the duck and the human. The other low pathogenic hosts of IAV are cat, horse, dog, ferret, seal, and whale. The subtypes of IAVs responsible for causing influenza in their host are also mentioned.

cats, pigs, horses, ferrets, seals, and whales (**Figure 1**). Avian IAV such as H5N1 and H9N2 are known to cause bird flu, whereas H1N1 and H3N2 are responsible for swine flu. IAVs are also categorized as seasonal and pandemic based on genetic variation and the severity of influenza disease; IAV transmission occurs by direct or indirect contact, inhaling virus-infected droplets or small droplet nuclei, being exposed to diseased poultry, feeding raw or undercooked poultry, transplacental transmission, or drinking water contaminated by viruses [7]. The serological evidence validated that human-to-human transmission of influenza viruses is inefficient; however, in some rare cases human-to-human transmission was observed during an outbreak of the highly pathogenic avian influenza viruses (HPAI) of H5N1 [8]. Influenza virus enters the human body through the respiratory tract and its incubation period is 1–7 days. The common symptoms associated with influenza are respiratory distress, fever, headache, cold, abdominal pain and joint pain [9]. With the progression of the disease, other symptoms observed are bloody sputum and pneumonia that further cause respiratory failure leading to acute respiratory distress syndrome (ARDS) [10]. IAV-infected patients can be diagnosed by reverse transcription-polymerase chain reaction (RT-PCR), viral culture, and the high levels of HA antigen- specific neutralizing antibodies.

3. Life cycle of influenza A virus

The IAV enters in the host cell by binding with surface receptors possessing sialic acid moiety. Viruses are internalized by endocytosis and the uncoating of the virus by matrix protein 2, an ion channel. The vRNA is released in the cytoplasm and is imported to the nucleus where vRNA is transcribed and replicated by using its polymerase [11]. Thus, these steps lead to the synthesis of a positive sense complementary RNA (cRNA) and viral messenger RNA (vmRNA) with 5′cap and 3′ poly (A) tail. The influenza virus polymerase does not exhibit capping activity at the 5′end; hence, they have to depend on host-capped mRNAs where they capture its 5′cap, a process known as cap snatching [12]. The viral m-RNA is translated in the cytoplasm after being exported from the nucleus and viral proteins, and nucleoproteins are synthesized by cellular ribosomes. Translated viral proteins re-enter the nucleus and bind to the vRNAs to generate viral ribonucleoproteins (vRNPs). Following nuclear export, progeny vRNPs and viral proteins are assembled to form virions which later egress from the host cell.

4. Pandemics and outbreaks of human influenza A virus

The prominent IAVs causing pandemics and outbreaks in various parts of the world are shown in the **Figures 2** and **3**, respectively. The 1918 spread of human influenza A(H1N1) virus has caused death of approximately 40–50 million people worldwide. This virus had again emerged in 2009 and caused a death toll of 4100 people. The clinical presentations were similar to the earlier strain that led to a less severe response. The twenty-first-century influenza viruses that cause infections in humans are briefly discussed below.

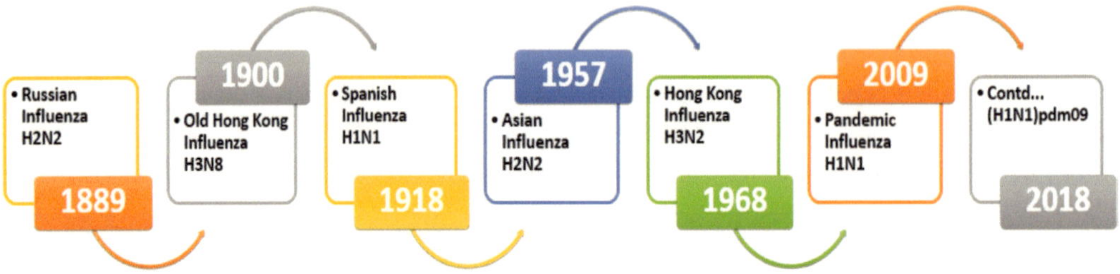

Figure 2. The pandemics of influenza A viruses. Noted influenza A virus pandemics are shown in the figure till 2018.

4.1. Influenza A(H5N1) virus

The first outbreak of human infection due to influenza A(H5N1) virus occurred in Hong Kong in 1997 with 18 cases and 6 deaths, following its re-emergence in regions of Southeast Asia during 2003, where 392 individuals were infected and 247 fatal outcomes were reported [13].

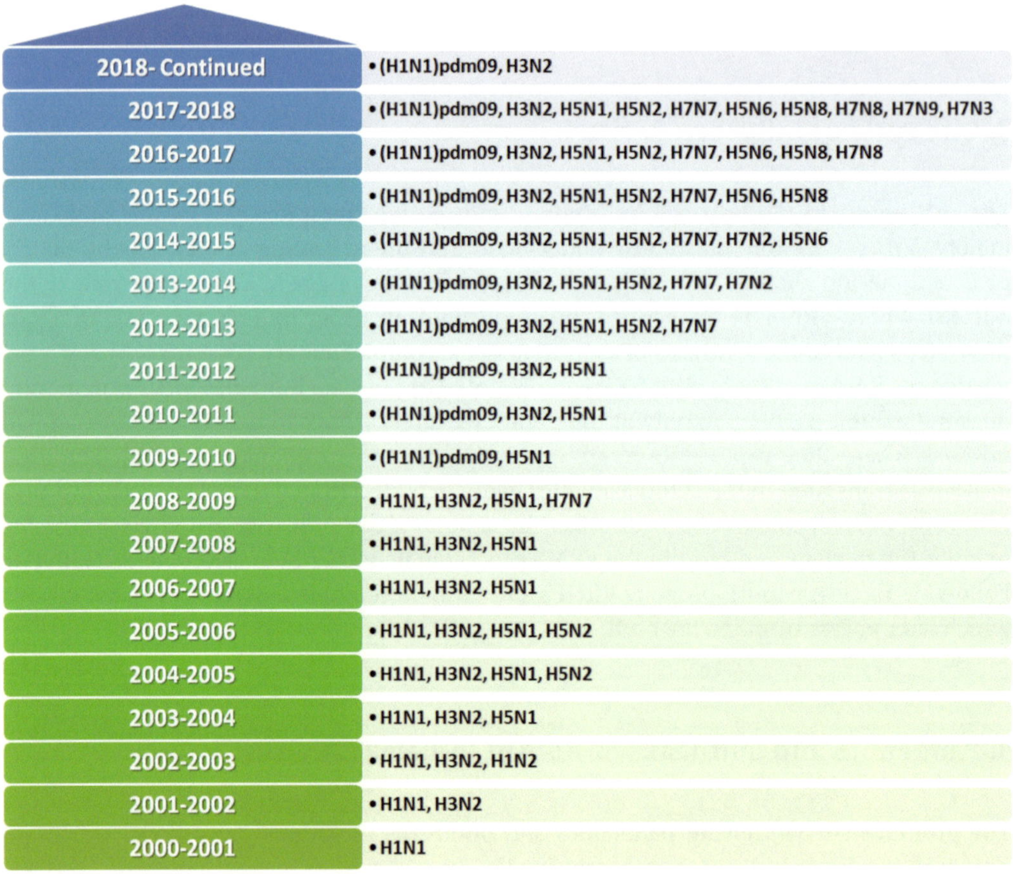

2018- Continued
• (H1N1)pdm09, H3N2
2017-2018
• (H1N1)pdm09, H3N2, H5N1, H5N2, H7N7, H5N6, H5N8, H7N8, H7N9, H7N3
2016-2017
• (H1N1)pdm09, H3N2, H5N1, H5N2, H7N7, H5N6, H5N8, H7N8
2015-2016
• (H1N1)pdm09, H3N2, H5N1, H5N2, H7N7, H5N6, H5N8
2014-2015
• (H1N1)pdm09, H3N2, H5N1, H5N2, H7N7, H7N2, H5N6
2013-2014
• (H1N1)pdm09, H3N2, H5N1, H5N2, H7N7, H7N2
2012-2013
• (H1N1)pdm09, H3N2, H5N1, H5N2, H7N7
2011-2012
• (H1N1)pdm09, H3N2, H5N1
2010-2011
• (H1N1)pdm09, H3N2, H5N1
2009-2010
• (H1N1)pdm09, H5N1
2008-2009
• H1N1, H3N2, H5N1, H7N7
2007-2008
• H1N1, H3N2, H5N1
2006-2007
• H1N1, H3N2, H5N1
2005-2006
• H1N1, H3N2, H5N1, H5N2
2004-2005
• H1N1, H3N2, H5N1, H5N2
2003-2004
• H1N1, H3N2, H5N1
2002-2003
• H1N1, H3N2, H1N2
2001-2002
• H1N1, H3N2
2000-2001
• H1N1

Figure 3. Recent outbreaks of influenza A virus in humans. The prominent influenza A viruses of twenty-first century causing most number of cases are shown in the picture.

This HPAI H5N1 virus further infected humans as well as migratory birds. The reported mortality rate was ~60% of the infected human population [14] and ~6000 deaths of migratory birds have been reported in Western China [15, 16].

4.2. Influenza A(H1N1)pdm09 virus

The first human infection from pandemic influenza A(H1N1)2009 virus was reported in Mexico and the United States in March 2009, and later it was transmitted globally [17]. The number of cases reported worldwide to the WHO in the period from March to September 2009 was 340,000 with 4100 deaths. In India, influenza A(H1N1)2009 was the pandemic, with 10,036 laboratory-reported cases and 308 deaths. The susceptible age groups infected were children of age less than 5 years and adults of more than 65 years, while pregnant women were at high risk of infection [18].

4.3. Influenza A(H7N9) virus

A highly pathogenic novel strain of IAV is H7N9, first reported in China in 2013. The Chinese Center for Disease Control and Prevention (China CDC) has actively investigated the first 82 patients infected with influenza A(H7N9) in the provinces of China [19] where the number of reported cases was 131 with 32 deaths. Based on the weekly report on April 20, 2017, the WHO has identified 1393 laboratory-observed cases of H7N9 virus with 534 deaths. Further, the WHO has assessed that within 2 months of the H7N9 outbreak, the number of cases were as many as of H5N1 in 10 years and till date cases of H7N9 are reported [20].

5. Immunobiology

Influenza viruses enter in humans through the respiratory tract by the oral or nasal route and the first barrier for the virus is to cross the mucous layer surrounding the respiratory epithelium. Then, through the mucous layer, influenza virus has to attach and internalize these epithelial cells to cause infection. The host defense mechanism is activated to prohibit the spread of the virus. Thus, the pattern recognition receptors (PRRs) detect the pathogen-associated molecular patterns (PAMPs) of the infectious viral agents and activate the host's innate immune system by the secretion of type-I interferons, pro-inflammatory cytokines and chemokines [21]. Respiratory tract cells such as macrophages, dendritic cells (DCs), pneumocytes and plasmacytoid DCs (pDCs) actively participate in production of type-I interferons that stimulates a pool of genes called interferon-stimulated genes (ISGs) (mentioned in **Table 1**) which enhance the antiviral activity of host defense system [22, 23]. These PRRs include the toll-like receptors such as TLR3 that recognizes the viral dsRNA present in infected cells; TLR7 and TLR8 detect viral ssRNA present in endosomes of infected cells; retinoic acid-inducible gene I (RIG-I) recognizes the virus present in the cytosol of infected cells [24]. The human respiratory epithelial cells constitutively express TLR3 that induces the generation of pro-inflammatory cytokines on the detection of influenza virus that stimulates the infiltration of leukocytes and CD8+ T cells restricting virus replication [25]. These

Interferon-stimulated genes (ISGs)	Intracellular location	Mode of action
Cholesterol 25-hydroxylase ($CH_{25}H$)	Cytosol	Inhibits fusion of virus with host cell membrane
2'-5'-Oligoadenylate synthase (OAS) and RNase L	Cytosol	Stimulates cleavage of viral RNA
Protein kinase R (PKR)	Cytosol	Inhibits translation and activates downstream NF-κB pathway
ISG15	Cytosol	Ubiquitin-like protein that targets newly translated viral proteins for modification
Tripartite motif-containing protein 22 (TRIM22)	Nucleus	Binds with nucleocapsid for proteasomal degradation
MX1	Nucleus	Inhibits viral transcription in nucleus
IFITM3 and other IFN-inducible transmembrane (IFITM) proteins	Endosomes	Inhibits viral attachment, fusion and endocytosis
Viperin	Lipid droplets and the cytosolic face of the endoplasmic reticulum	Inhibits egression of virus by blocking formation of the lipid raft

Table 1. Role of pertinent interferon-stimulated genes (ISG) in controlling influenza virus infection (adapted from Ref. [4]).

pro-inflammatory cytokines cause local inflammation and fever that activate the adaptive immune response against influenza virus. Chemokines instruct downstream immune cells by recruiting neutrophils, monocytes and natural killer (NK) cells to the respiratory tract. NK cells target and eliminate the virus-infected epithelial cells initiating viral clearance [26]. Monocytes and neutrophils participate in the removal of dead cells infected with virus. Alveolar macrophages cause the phagocytic clearance of infected cells, a crucial step for virus clearance [27]. The innate and adaptive immune system works hand in hand for the clearance of the influenza virus from the host system.

6. Antiviral therapeutics

Numerous antiviral drugs inhibiting influenza viruses are available. The most targeted sites for restricting influenza viruses are matrix protein 2 and NA, inhibited by antivirals such as adamantanes (amantadine and rimantadine), oseltamivir, and zanamivir [28]. The adamantanes interfere with viral uncoating and had shown toxic effects that lead to the generation of adamantanes-resistant strains of the influenza virus. Furthermore, the budding off progeny virions from host cells is impeded by the neuraminidase inhibitors that caused only one round of replication, hence preventing the spread of infection. Influenza viruses such as influenza A(H3N2) and A(H1N1)pdm09 were observed to be resistant for adamantanes; therefore, for the clinical treatment of influenza virus A, adamantanes are not recommended. However, IAV and influenza B virus are susceptible to oseltamivir and zanamivir [29]. The other potential targeted sites are viral entry, HA, pH-dependent endosomal fusion, nucleoproteins and polymerase proteins of influenza viruses. HA1 and HA2 play key roles in the invasion of the influenza virus in target host cells. HA1 binds with the sialic acid receptors while HA2 contributes in the fusion and internalization by endocytosis. Furthermore, a novel antiviral N-stearoyllipopeptide of C18-ARLPR inhibits the viral replication of influenza A/Puerto Rico/8/34 (H1N1) and A/Aichi/2/68 (H3N2) effectively with low toxicity [30]. This peptide adequately binds to the sialic acid-binding site of HA1 subunit due to its structural similarity.

7. Complementary and alternative medicine (CAM)

The National Centre for Complementary and Integrative Health-National Institute of Health (NCCIH-NIH), the United States, describes complementary and alternative medicine (CAM) as a collection of varied medicinal practices, natural products, and health-care systems, different from conventional medicine [31]. CAMs treat the disease effectively with fewer side effects and low toxicity [32]. Several plant products are globally applied for the treatment of influenza, though the mechanism of their action is still unknown. The extracts of plants are prepared at very high dilution and are given in small doses. The interaction of active components of plant extracts and viral proteins of the influenza virus is further explored for discovering a potent organic antiviral against a pandemic virus such as H1N1. Some of the reported natural compounds for the treatment of human influenza are baicalin, tinosporon, allicin, curcumin, ursolic acid, carvacrol, ajoene, methanol, andrographolide, coumarin, theaflavin, and eugenol [33]. In *in silico* study, these natural compounds blocked H1N1 NA effectively with significant values of binding energies. Several traditional plants such as *Trachyspermum ammi, Ocimum sanctum, Zingiber officinalis, Allium sativum, Curcuma longa, Tinospora cordifolia,* and *Mentha piperita* are potential antiviral agents against H1N1 swine flu. Another plant-based antiviral agent, ginseng (*Panax quinquefolium*), has triterpenes and saponins that are the potent inhibitors of influenza A(H1N1) pdm09 [34]. The CAM therapies for the treatment of influenza virus also include influenzinum that induces cytokine release from macrophages and furthermore activates the innate immune response [3]. In a study, IAV H3N2-infected MDCK cells were treated with influenzinum and it was observed that there was no cytotoxic effect due to influenzinum, yet the morphology of cells were altered [35].

8. Prevention and control

The transmission of influenza virus between humans and other hosts like avian and swine was reported to be possible and significantly caused pandemics in various countries [36]. The viruses responsible for infecting humans are HPAI or low-pathogenicity avian influenza (LPAI) viruses. Owing to the enormous ability of re-assortment (due to shift and drift) in influenza viruses, absolute prediction of the responsible subtype(s) for the next pandemic infection is impractical. Thus, a vaccine which can effectively target a broad range of influenza viruses is required for the protection of the human host. The development of the vaccine should be dependent on several strategies such as epidemiological data of the previous pandemic influenza viruses, the presence of viruses in nature, and viruses responsible for infecting human population. The current influenza vaccines are live-attenuated influenza vaccines (LAIV), influenza-inactivated vaccine (IIV), recombinant subunit, DNA and vectored virus vaccine [37]. According to Centers for Disease Control and

Prevention (CDCs), the United States, available vaccines are of two types—trivalent and quadrivalent flu vaccines. Trivalent influenza vaccine protects against influenza A(H1N1) and A(H3N2) as well as influenza B virus. The standard-dose trivalent flu shots are IIV 3, given to individuals between 18 and 64 years. The CDC has not recommended using LAIV as the vaccines for the year 2017–2018 due to its low effectiveness found during 2013–2017. There are some limitations associated with influenza virus vaccines suggesting that the circulating virus and the vaccine virus should be of same strains to give a high efficacy or else the vaccine might provide a false sense of security. The early influenza vaccination of individuals at a high risk might prevent influenza from becoming a pandemic. The Advisory Committee on Immunization Practices (ACIP) has recommended to primarily providing vaccination to children, pregnant women, individuals of age more than 65 years, and to people suffering from chronic ailments [38]. The other effective methods to control influenza are properly washing hands, use of masks, and covering mouth during coughing and sneezing, avoiding physical contacts with influenza-infected individuals, wearing gloves while working with infected poultry or swine, and the intake of effective antiviral medications.

9. Conclusions and future perspectives

Several factors play a pivotal role in preventing influenza virus infection such as increasing antigenic and genetic variants of influenza virus subtypes, the ability to cross the species barrier, antiviral drug resistance, incapability in predicting the upcoming pandemic virus, the low probability of correctly matching the circulating and vaccine viruses, and the high cost of vaccination. Thus, a robust surveillance system that monitors the human influenza viruses will provide the candidate virus vaccine (CVV) as an adequate strategy required for preparing the pandemics. Apart from this, a comprehensive understanding at the molecular and genetic level of the avian and swine influenza virus will strengthen us in understanding their mechanism of re-assortment and transmission in humans. The veterinary vaccines designed for avian and swine population should be examined to evaluate their efficacy on the avian and swine influenza viruses. Furthermore, there is a crucial requirement of the universal vaccine that can target both seasonal and pandemic influenza viruses. Awareness regarding the prevention and control methods of influenza should be widely spread.

Acknowledgements

The authors are grateful to the Vice Chancellor, King George's Medical University (KGMU), Lucknow, and Director, Centre for Cellular and Molecular Biology, Council of Scientific and Industrial Research (CSIR-CCMB), India, for the encouragement and support for this work. SK Saxena is also supported by CCRH, the Government of India, and US NIH grants: R37DA025576 and R01MH085259. The authors have no other relevant affiliations or financial involvement with any organization or entity with a financial interest or financial conflict with the subject matter or materials discussed in the manuscript apart from those disclosed.

Author details

Shailendra K. Saxena[1,2]*, Amrita Haikerwal[1], Swatantra Kumar[1] and Madan L.B. Bhatt[1]

*Address all correspondence to: myedrsaxena@gmail.com

1 Centre for Advance Research, King George's Medical University, Lucknow, India

2 CSIR-Centre for Cellular and Molecular Biology (CCMB), Hyderabad, India

References

[1] World Health Organization. Influenza Update No. 312: Summary. April 2018. Available from: http://www.who.int/influenza/surveillance_monitoring/updates/2018_04_02_surveillance_update_312.pdf?ua=1 [Accessed: April 16, 2018]

[2] World Health Organization. Influenza (Seasonal). Fact Sheet. January 2018. Available from: http://www.who.int/mediacentre/factsheets/fs211/en [Accessed: April 16, 2018]

[3] Ferhadian D, Contrant M, Printz-Schweigert A, Smyth RP, Paillart JC, Marquet R. Structural and functional motifs in influenza virus RNAs. Frontiers in Microbiology. 2018;**9**:559-570

[4] Iwasaki A, Pillai PS. Innate immunity to influenza virus infection. Nature Reviews. Immunology. 2014;**14**(5):315-328

[5] Krammer F, Palese P. Advances in the development of influenza virus vaccines. Nature Reviews. Drug Discovery. 2015;**14**(3):167-182

[6] Petrova VN, Russell CA. The evolution of seasonal influenza viruses. Nature Reviews. Microbiology. 2018;**16**(1):60-74

[7] Beigel JH, Farrar J, Han AM, Hayden FG, Hyer R, de Jong MD, Lochindarat S, Nguyen TK, Nguyen TH, Tran TH, Nicoll A, Touch S, Yuen KY, Writing Committee of the World Health Organization (WHO). Consultation on human influenza A/H5. Avian influenza A (H5N1) infection in humans. The New England Journal of Medicine. 2005;**353**(13):1374-1385

[8] Ungchusak K, Auewarakul P, Dowell SF, Kitphati R, Auwanit W, Puthavathana P, Uiprasertkul M, Boonnak K, Pittayawonganon C, Cox NJ, Zaki SR, Thawatsupha P, Chittaganpitch M, Khontong R, Simmerman JM, Chunsutthiwat S. Probable person-to-person transmission of avian influenza A (H5N1). The New England Journal of Medicine. 2005;**352**(4):333-340

[9] Saxena SK, Kotikalapudi R, Tiwari S, Muvva C. Influenz A(H1N1)pdm09 virus: Therapeutics and challenges. Future Virology. 2012;**7**(10):947-950

[10] Chotpitayasunondh T, Ungchusak K, Hanshaoworakul W, Chunsuthiwat S, Sawanpanyalert P, Kijphati R, Lochindarat S, Srisan P, Suwan P, Osotthanakorn Y, Anan tasetagoon T, Kanjanawasri S, Tanupattarachai S, Weerakul J, Chaiwirattana R, Manee

rattanaporn M, Poolsavathitikool R, Chokephaibulkit K, Apisarnthanarak A, Dowell SF. Human disease from influenza A (H5N1), Thailand, 2004. Emerging Infectious Diseases. 2005;**11**(2):201-209

[11] TeVelthuis AJ, Fodor E. Influenza virus RNA polymerase: Insights into the mechanisms of viral RNA synthesis. Nature Reviews. Microbiology. 2016;**14**(8):479-493

[12] Guilligay D, Tarendeau F, Resa-Infante P, Coloma R, Crepin T, Sehr P, Lewis J, Ruigrok RW, Ortin J, Hart DJ, Cusack S. The structural basis for cap binding by influenza virus polymerase subunit PB2. Nature Structural & Molecular Biology. 2008;**15**(5):500-506

[13] Neumann G, Chen H, Gao GF, Shu Y, Kawaoka Y. H5N1 influenza viruses: Outbreaks and biological properties. Cell Research. 2010;**20**(1):51-61

[14] World Health Organization. H5N1 Influenza. 2017. Available from: http://www.who.int/influenza/human_animal_interface/avian_influenza/h5n1_research/faqs/en/ [Accessed: April 16, 2018]

[15] Chen H, Li Y, Li Z, Shi J, Shinya K, Deng G, Qi Q, Tian G, Fan S, Zhao H, Sun Y, Kawaoka Y. Properties and dissemination of H5N1 viruses isolated during aninfluenza outbreak in migratory waterfowl in western China. Journal of Virology. 2006;**80**(12):5976-5983

[16] Liu J, Xiao H, Lei F, Zhu Q, Qin K, Zhang XW, Zhang XL, Zhao D, Wang G, Feng Y, Ma J, Liu W, Wang J, Gao GF. Highly pathogenic H5N1 influenza virus infection in migratory birds. Science. 2005;**309**(5738):1206

[17] Neumann G, Noda T, Kawaoka Y. Emergence and pandemic potential of swine-origin H1N1 influenza virus. Nature. 2009;**459**(7249):931-939

[18] Pandemic Influenza Virus (H1N1)2009. National Centre for disease control. CD Alert. 2009;**13**(2):1-8

[19] Li Q, Zhou L, Zhou M, Chen Z, Li F, Wu H, Xiang N, Chen E, Tang F, Wang D,Meng L, Hong Z, Tu W, Cao Y, Li L, Ding F, Liu B, Wang M, Xie R, Gao R, Li X, Bai T, Zou S, He J, Hu J, Xu Y, Chai C, Wang S, Gao Y, Jin L, Zhang Y, Luo H, Yu H,He J, Li Q, Wang X, Gao L, Pang X, Liu G, Yan Y, Yuan H, Shu Y, Yang W, Wang Y, Wu F, Uyeki TM, Feng Z. Epidemiology of human infections with avian influenza A(H7N9) virus in China. The New England Journal of Medicine. 2014;**370**(6):520-532

[20] World Health Organization. Avian influenza A (H7N9) virus. 2017. Available from: http://www.who.int/influenza/human_animal_interface/influenza_h7n9/en/ [Accessed: April 16, 2018]

[21] Medzhitov R. Toll-like receptors and innate immunity. Nature Reviews Immunology. 2001;**1**(2):135-145

[22] Högner K, Wolff T, Pleschka S, Plog S, Gruber AD, Kalinke U, Walmrath HD, Bodner J, Gattenlöhner S, Lewe-Schlosser P, Matrosovich M, Seeger W, Lohmeyer J, Herold S. Macrophage-expressed IFN-β contributes to apoptotic alveolar epithelialcell injury in severe influenza virus pneumonia. PLoS Pathogens. 2013;**9**(2):e1003188

[23] Kallfass C, Lienenklaus S, Weiss S, Staeheli P. Visualizing the betainterferon response in mice during infection with influenza A viruses expressing or lacking nonstructural protein 1. Journal of Virology. 2013;**87**(12):6925-6930

[24] Pang IK, Iwasaki A. Control of antiviral immunity by pattern recognition and the microbiome. Immunological Reviews. 2012;**245**(1):209-226

[25] Le Goffic R, Balloy V, Lagranderie M, Alexopoulou L, Escriou N, Flavell R, Chignard M, Si-Tahar M. Detrimental contribution of the toll-like receptor (TLR)3 to influenza A virus-induced acute pneumonia. PLoS Pathogens. 2006;**2**(6):e53

[26] Gazit R, Gruda R, Elboim M, Arnon TI, Katz G, Achdout H, Hanna J, Qimron U, Landau G, Greenbaum E, Zakay-Rones Z, Porgador A, Mandelboim O. Lethal influenza infection in the absence of the natural killer cell receptor gene Ncr1. Nature Immunology. 2006;**7**(5):517-523

[27] Hashimoto Y, Moki T, Takizawa T, Shiratsuchi A, Nakanishi Y. Evidence forphagocytosis of influenza virus-infected, apoptotic cells by neutrophils andmacrophages in mice. Journal of Immunology. 2007;**178**(4):2448-2457

[28] Moscona A. Neuraminidase inhibitors for influenza. The New England Journal of Medicine. 2005;**353**(13):1363-1373

[29] Centers for Disease Control and Prevention, National Center for Immunization and Respiratory Diseases (NCIRD). Weekly U.S. Influenza Surveillance Report. 2018. Available from: http://www.cdc.gov/flu/weekly [Accessed: April 16, 2018]

[30] Lin D, Li F, Wu Q, Xie X, Wu W, Wu J, Chen Q, Liu S, He J. A "building block" approach to the new influenza A virus entry inhibitors with reduced cellular toxicities. Scientific Reports. 2016;**6**(3):22790

[31] National Center for Complementary and Integrative Health (NCCIH). Complementary, Alternative, or Integrative Health: What's In a Name? U.S. Department of Health & Human Services, National Institutes of Health. Available from: https://nccih.nih.gov/health/integrative-health [Accessed: April 16, 2018]

[32] Saxena SK, Chitti SV, Gadugu S. Complementary and alternative medicine in alliance with conventional medicine for influenza therapeutics and prevention. Future Virology. 2016;**11**(10):661-664

[33] Sahoo M, Jena L, Rath SN, Kumar S. Identification of suitable natural inhibitor against influenza A (H1N1) neuraminidase protein by molecular docking. Genomics & Informatics. 2016;**14**(3):96-103

[34] Dong W, Farooqui A, Leon AJ, Kelvin DJ. Inhibition of influenza A virus infection by ginsenosides. PLoS One. 2017;**12**(2):1-13

[35] Holandino C, Veiga V, Barbosa GM, Homsani F, Siqueira CM, Galina A, El-Bacha T, Couceiro JN, Luis Souza dos Santos A. Homeopathic medicines influences fungal adhesion and cellular oxygen metabolism of MDCK and MA104 cell lines. International Journal of High Dilution Research. 2014;**13**(47):97-98

[36] Lewis DB. Avian flu to human influenza. Annual Review of Medicine. 2006;**57**(2):139-154

[37] Subbarao K, Joseph T. Scientific barriers to developing vaccines against avian influenza viruses. Nature Reviews. Immunology. 2007;**7**(4):267-278

[38] Grohskopf LA, Sokolow LZ, Broder KR, Walter EB, Bresee JS, Fry AM, Jernigan DB. Prevention and control of seasonal influenza with vaccines: Recommendations of the advisory committee on immunization practices – United States, 2017-18 influenza season. MMWR – Recommendations and Reports. 2017;**66**(2):1-20

Section 2

Pathogenesis of Influenza

Chapter 2

Pathology of Influenza

Vsevolod A. Zinserling

Additional information is available at the end of the chapter

http://dx.doi.org/10.5772/intechopen.76309

Abstract

The chapter is based upon the own experience of scientific school the author belongs in comparison with the published data. Special attention is paid to three types of cellular changes related to viral replication, immediate causes of death, extrapulmonary lesions, and peculiarities of lesions in experimental mice model. Different courses of the disease and morphologic appearance during different epidemics are analyzed as well.

Keywords: influenza, histopathology, immediate death causes

1. Introduction

Influenza A and influenza B can present along a broad spectrum of disease, ranging from subclinical to severe generalized infection leading to numerous lethal outcomes causing pandemia and epidemics or developing as sporadic cases [1]. Particular attention of clinicians, physicians, virologists, and molecular biologists, as well as public media, is devoted to the lesions of respiratory organs during the epidemics with most severe course of the disease. Only in clinical practice such cases usually are officially registered as influenza. Pathological studies are much less in number and usually devoted only to changes in the trachea and lungs in single cases or small series of autopsy observations. In majority of manuals, pathology in influenza is characterized as vascular disorders or viral pneumonia [2, 3]. No typical changes related to virus replication are discussed. The data related to histopathological changes in extrapulmonary lesions are very scarce in spite of widely accepted fact that influenza negatively influences upon the course of myocardial infarction and other forms of ischemic heart disease. It has been considered for a long time that the most severe illness with possible lethal outcomes usually develops in infants and elderly persons due to decreased immune reactions. In 2009–2011 during the epidemics caused by H1N1 virus (so-called swine strain) all over the world, the most of lethal outcomes occurred in middle-age patients with the signs of metabolic syndrome, but this fact has not been explained in the literature [4–9]. The fact that influenza has more severe course in pregnant women has been described by many authors [10], but its pathogenesis remains unclear. In the literature, one cannot find special analysis of immediate death causes related to different periods of time, virus strains, and age of the deceased.

In Saint Petersburg/Leningrad (Russia, former Soviet Union), pathology of influenza has been studied by Zinserling (Tsinzerling) (1923–1995), his collaborators, and pupils since the end of 60th. The most of numerous publications of that time were in Russia, partly summarized in monographs and manuals [11], but he succeeded to make several contributions in the world literature as well [12, 13]. The most significant data received at that time was demonstration of typical cell changes, called by him "influenza cells." Cytoplasm enlarged being at early stages of the disease basophilic, later on parallel with virus disappearance pale stained and showing signs of degeneration. Intracytoplasmic fuchsinophilic inclusions were considered as very typical, although not specific, for influenza, representing the necrotic foci surrounded by the membrane. Appearing as small dots in the perinuclear zones, they grew in size and were transferred at the periphery being expelled afterward. Such transformations were observed in ciliated epithelial cells of the trachea and bronchi, alveolocytes, and lung macrophages. As exception such inclusions were noted also in smears from meninges and placenta. In infants and small children basing upon clinical, virological data and immunofluorescent microscopy, generalized infection was proven in many cases with development of brain, liver, kidney, intestine, and adrenal lesions partly with appearance of "influenza cells." In adults the majority of lethal cases were explained by bacterial, at that time usually staphylococcal, superinfection leading to destructive pneumonias. Mucous layer in the larynx, trachea and bronchi was swollen with mixed infiltration and desquamation of epithelium. Viral antigen could also be detected in capillary endothelium. Described changes were found in all cases of influenza due to viruses H3N2 and B, regardless of its clinical manifestation. In cases with expressed clinical symptoms, lung edemas and plethora of vessels with hemorrhagic foci were observed. Neutrophilic infiltration was considered as a hallmark of bacterial superinfection. Indeed, in majority of cases of focal pneumonias, viral-bacterial associations have been found. Bacterial pneumonia can be both community and hospital acquired.

Later on the progress of clinical and preventive medicine resulted in critical decrease of lethal outcomes due to influenza. Situation changed with appearance of the new "swine" strain of virus. Our new experience was partly summarized in Russian [14, 15] and international press [16].

Pathomorphological features and disease severity depend on patient general state and susceptibility, as well as the virus type in question. The so-called H1N1 avian influenza virus is considered to be the most dangerous virus, causing generalized infection with more than 50% lethality. Seasonal H3N2 and H1N1 influenza viruses that have been circulating in recent years tend to cause primarily localized respiratory infection, although extrapulmonary lesions may occur in severe cases. New H1N1 influenza virus also causes mainly localized infection, but in most autopsies, signs of generalization can be found. Also, it should be noted that bacterial coinfections are relatively rare.

Diagnosis is based upon the epidemiological, clinical, and virological data. At the autopsy enlarged slightly firmed reddish lungs were very typical (**Figure 1**), while in histological examination, the changes of the infected cells becoming enlarged intensively stained cytoplasm were very informative. In other respiratory infections, either cytoproliferative changes (respiratory-syncytial and parainfluenza) or intranuclear basophilic inclusion (adenoviral and respiratory herpes) is notified.

Our experience based upon about thousand observations in the period 1977–2017 allows us to make several not widely known statements:

1. Clinical course of influenza may differ, and sometimes, usually in intraepidemic periods, the disease may manifest with moderate symptoms usual for all acute respiratory infections of different viral etiologies (rhinitis, cough, etc.).

2. Our data allow to confirm the existence of previously described in experiment chronic forms of influenza without distinct clinical symptoms, being able to be activated in unfavorable for the patient situation, superinfection by other pathogens first of all. Persistence of viral antigens in lung macrophages without signs of inflammation has been proven in our study with the help of immunohistochemistry (**Figure 2**). One can submit that this phenomenon has to be studied specially and can be considered in relation to survival of "not actual" viral strains. Once, we had the opportunity to detect such strain in plexus choroideus of 4.5 month girl.

3. It is widely accepted and properly investigated that all types and antigenic variants of influenza virus have tropism to ciliated epithelial cells of the trachea and bronchi of different calibers. In single publications it has been demonstrated that alveolocytes, lung macrophages, and endothelial cells can be considered as targets for virus as well (**Figure 3**). In accordance with our experience, virus-exposed cells are submitted to typical transformation which can differ due to properties of virus strain. During the infection caused by virus with short replicative period (H3N2 as example), one can observe during the first 3 days of the infection of the cells with the enlarged slightly basophilic cytoplasm ("influenza cells" of Zinserling) (**Figure 4**). Such changes were explained by active viral replication. Later on (5th–7th day

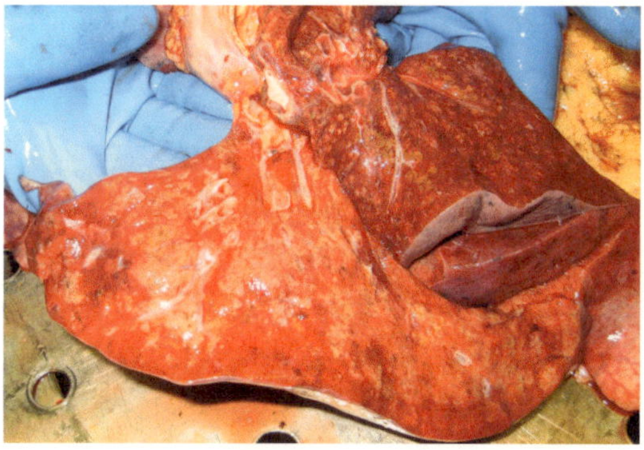

Figure 1. Macroscopic view of the lung of a deceased patient from influenza A H1N1 California pdm "swine".

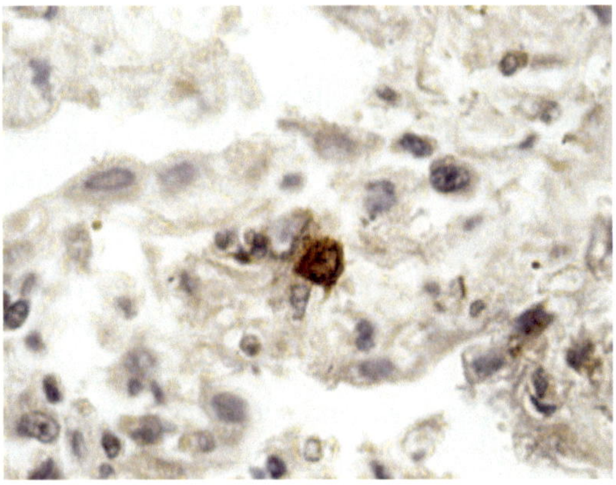

Figure 2. Antigen of influenza A virus nucleoprotein in cytoplasm of interstitial alveolar macrophages without any inflammatory changes in a patient without signs of respiratory infection (IHC, ×400).

of the disease), the cells are desquamated and undergo necrotic changes, which are hallmarked by cytoplasm becoming pale with indistinct cell borders. In the infection due to strains with prolonged virus replication in lungs (H1N1 California first of all), one can assume that virus-cell interactions undergo important modifications and the infected cells instead of dying express proliferative changes. In our experience they can become binucleated (**Figure 5**), considerably enlarged (**Figure 6**), multinucleated (**Figure 7**), or even undergo squamous cell metaplasia (**Figure 8**). Comparison between two types of cell changes due to influenza virus is presented in **Table 1**. From **Table 1** it is evident that recently described influenza cells of the two types typical for influenza H1N1 California are larger ($p \le 0,05$) than influenza cells described and studied by Zinserling and are distinguished from them also by larger nucleus-cytoplasm index ($p \le 0,05$). It is evident that the fine mechanisms of such only recently described phenomenon need further study.

4. In many lethal cases due to influenza, we deal with mixed infection. The most evident variant of its development is bacterial superinfection in the course of influenza leading to

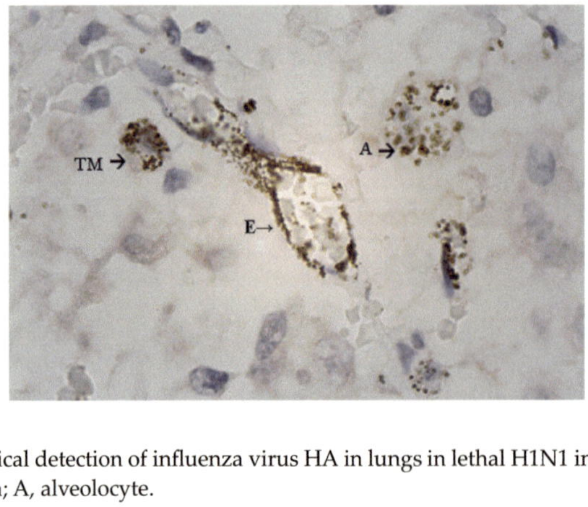

Figure 3. Immunohistochemical detection of influenza virus HA in lungs in lethal H1N1 influenza (×1000): TM, alveolar macrophage; Э, endothelium; A, alveolocyte.

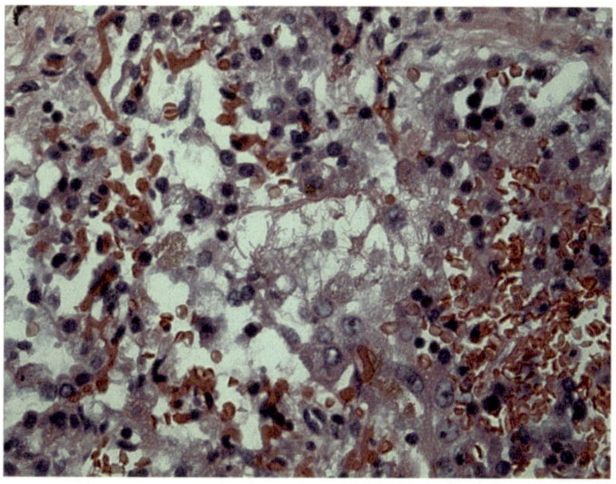

Figure 4. Lungs in lethal H1N1 influenza: the first type of virus-affected ("influenza") cells with prominent hyperemia and dystelectasis (H&E, ×400).

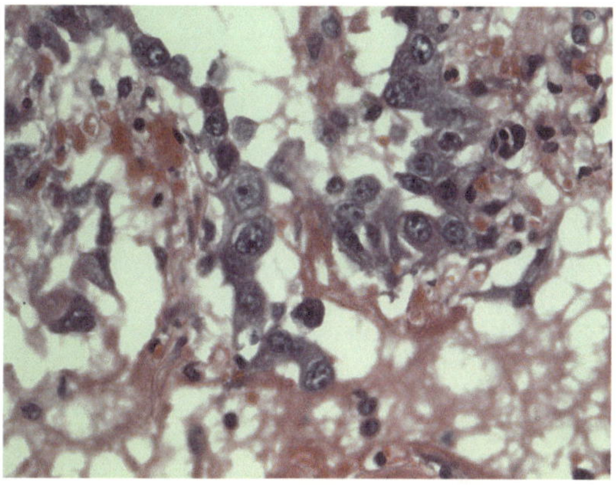

Figure 5. Lungs in lethal H1N1 influenza: the second type of virus-affected ("influenza") cells (H&E, ×600).

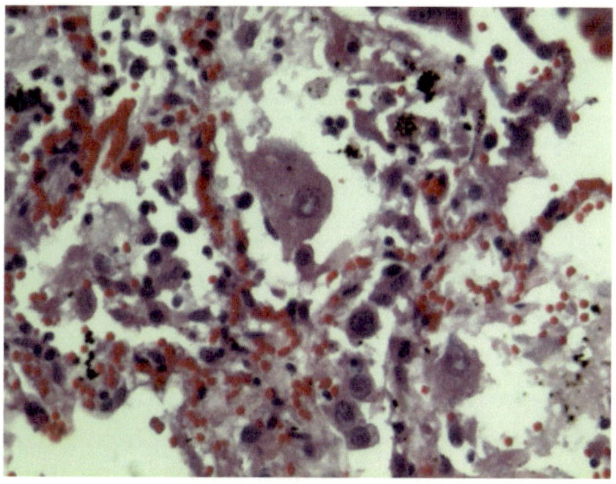

Figure 6. Enlarged alveolar macrophages (H&E, ×600).

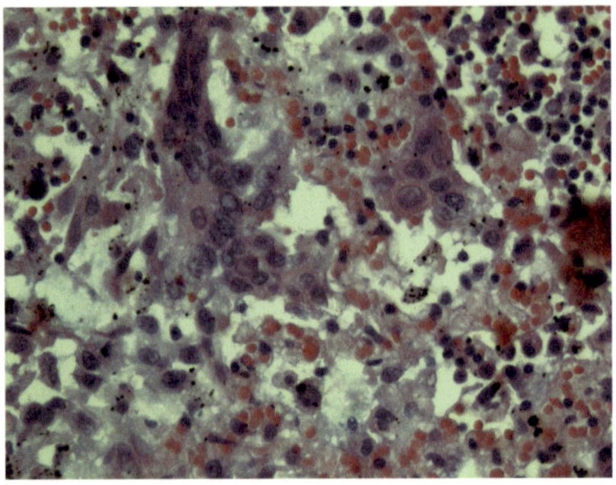

Figure 7. Giant multinuclear cells (H&E, ×600).

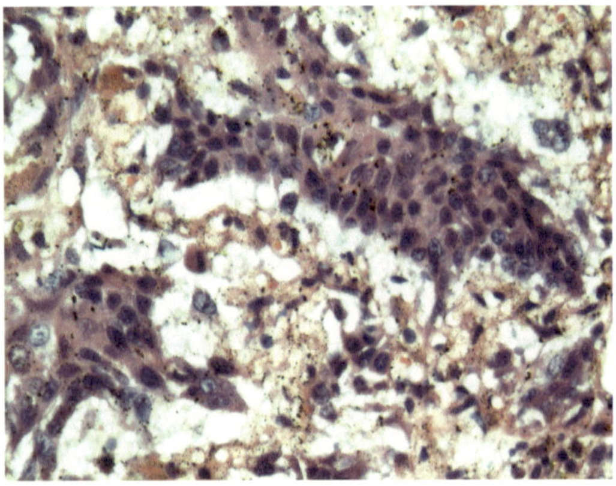

Figure 8. Squamous cell metaplasia (H&E, ×600).

	Influenza cells (first type)	Influenza cells (second type)
Square (relative unit)	14,273.6 ± 1099.8	19,715.3 ± 1436.4
Nucleus-cytoplasm index	0.274 ± 0.014	0.347 ± 0.016

Table 1. Square and nucleus-cytoplasm index in influenza cells of the first and second type ($n = 50$; $p < 0.05$).

defect of defense mechanisms of respiratory tract due to desquamation of ciliated cells. Later on viral-bacterial pneumonia develops playing an important role in clinical manifestations and tanatogenesis in lethal cases. Bacterial pneumonias are focal, usually confluent, frequently with signs of tissue destruction. The etiology of such bacterial superinfection can differ, in certain periods of time with prevalence of staphylococci, but in majority of cases stays undetermined either clinically or at the autopsy. Interestingly that during the lethal outcomes in 2009–2011 with the leading role in pathogenesis of diffuse alveolar damage (DAD), the expression of neutrophilic infiltration usually explained by bacterial component was rather modest. Certainly, this fact can partly be explained as a result of the efficacy of antibiotic treatment, but the same tendency was noted also in the patient without it.

Another case demonstrates practically not discussed in the literature variant of development of mixed infection is activation due to influenza virus influence of another preexisting, but not manifestating infection. One of our observations allows to suspect such possibility with high probability.

Case report of lethal influenza A/H1N1/California

One of the studied cases is of particular interest. We succeeded to provide more detailed investigation using immunohistochemical detection of *Chlamydia* spp., *Adenovirus*, influenza H1N1, *Herpes simplex* type 1 and type 2 (HSV1/HSV2), cytomegalovirus (CMV), Epstein–Barr virus (EBV), RSV, enterovirus, parvovirus, *Mycoplasma pneumoniae*, as well as electron microscopy. The latter was performed as follows: samples were fixated in glutaraldehyde 4 hours after death and then treated with osmium oxide, and uranyl acetate was used for contrast enhancement. Dehydration and embedding were performed using conventional techniques. Sections were analyzed on electron microscope JEM-100S.

A 31-year-old male patient IV with obesity got ill acutely, with fever up to 39°C. Three days later he was hospitalized to the intensive care unit with severe respiratory insufficiency. Intubation and, later on, tracheostomy were performed. The clinical diagnosis of "swine influenza" was supported by RT-PCR and serology (increase of the antibody level from 0 to 640). In spite of intensive treatment including antibiotics and antiviral drugs, the patient died on the 35th day of the illness.

Macroscopic changes. At the autopsy remarkable changes were found only in the lungs: necrotic posttracheostomic tracheitis, large abscesses in the lower lobes of the lungs in the stage of organization, and bilateral fibrinous pleuritis. The rest of the lung tissue was dark red and firm.

Microscopic changes. During the histological examination in the lungs, changes typical for rather old abscesses and late stages of respiratory distress syndrome were noted (**Figure 9**). The changes that we consider to be typical for influenza (virus-induced transformation of epithelial cells) were expressed only in the moderate number of the cells. We notified numerous intra-alveolar macrophages, partly with vacuolated cytoplasm (**Figure 10**), and PAS-positive inclusions. Some cells had slightly enlarged hyperchromic nuclei. Similar changes were noted in other organs as well.

Postmortem laboratory investigation. Postmortem RT-PCR of lung and spleen specimens for influenza A/H1N1sw was negative. During the bacteriological investigation of lung specimens, cultures of *E. coli*, nonpathogenic *Corynebacterium*, *Enterococcus*, *S. viridans*, and *S. epidermidis* were isolated.

Immunohistochemical investigation. In lungs strong positive reactions with serum against *Chlamydia* spp. (**Figure 11**), moderate against *Adenovirus* (**Figure 12**), and weak against influenza H1N1 were obtained. The reactions with sera against HSV1/2, CMV, EBV, RS, enterovirus, and parvoviruses, as well as *Mycoplasma pneumoniae*, were negative.

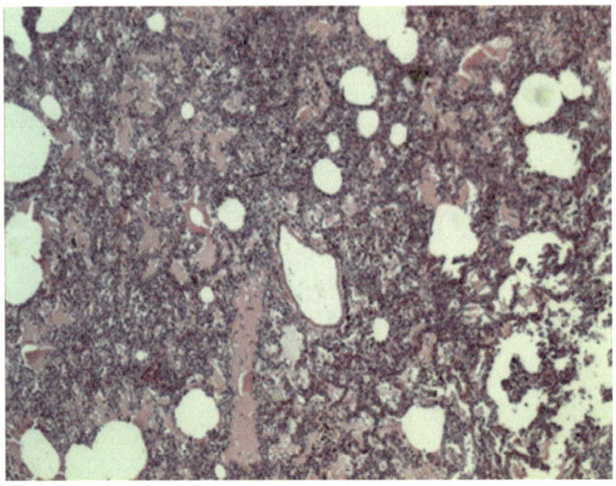

Figure 9. Lungs of a patient IV deceased from H1N1 influenza at low-power magnification, signs of moderate DAD (H&E, ×100).

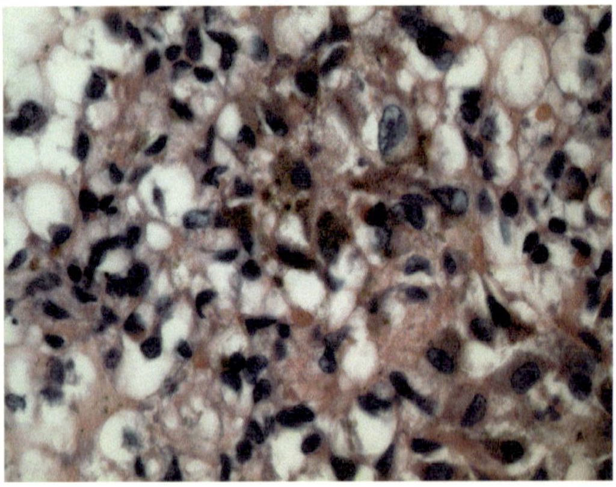

Figure 10. Lungs of the same patient, prevalence of macrophages in the exudate (H&E, ×640).

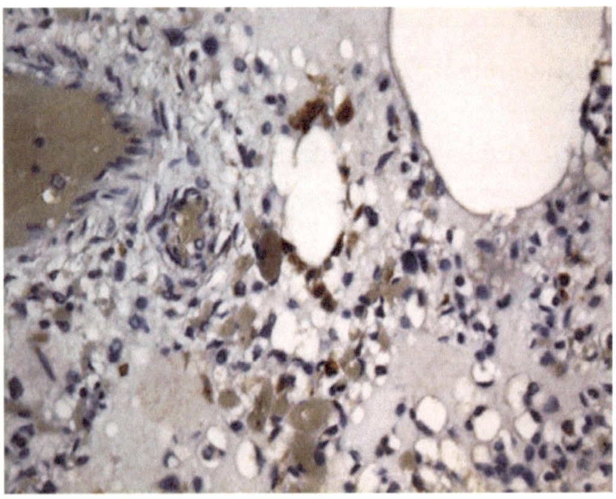

Figure 11. Lungs of the same patient, IHC with serum against *Chlamydia* spp. (×400).

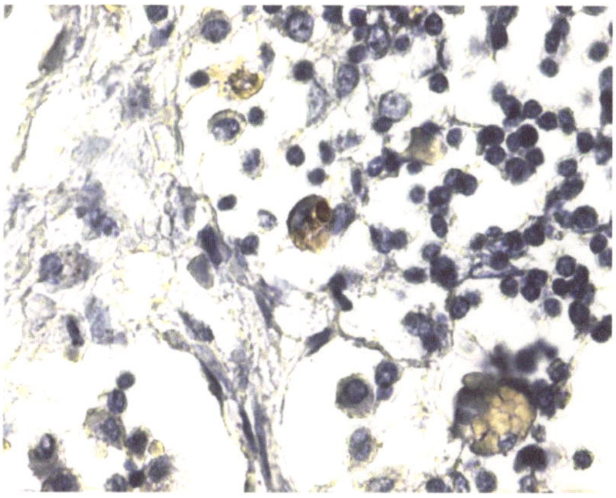

Figure 12. Lung lymph node of the same patient, IHC with serum against adenovirus (×640).

Electron microscopy. During the electron microscopic investigation of lungs, we succeeded to evaluate numerous elementary and reticular bodies of *Chlamydia* (**Figure 13**), in the brain only reticular bodies, predominantly in the cytoplasm of endothelial cells. In their nuclei several PML nuclear bodies (small intranucleolar inclusions containing promyelocytic leukemia protein) were found (**Figure 14**).

Conclusion. Death of a young previously healthy man occurred on the 35th day of illness clinically regarded as influenza with bacterial superinfection. The results of postmortem morphological and laboratory investigation proved that clinically diagnosed infections were expressed rather weakly but provoked the activation and severe course of respiratory chlamydiosis (with probable generalization) and adenoviral infection.

5. Practically, all authors from all over the world describing the lethal outcomes due to epidemic strain of influenza A virus underline the development of DAD syndrome with respiratory insufficiency resistant to treatment. During the postmortem morphological investigation macroscopically, firm reddish lungs vaguely resembling red congestion seen in

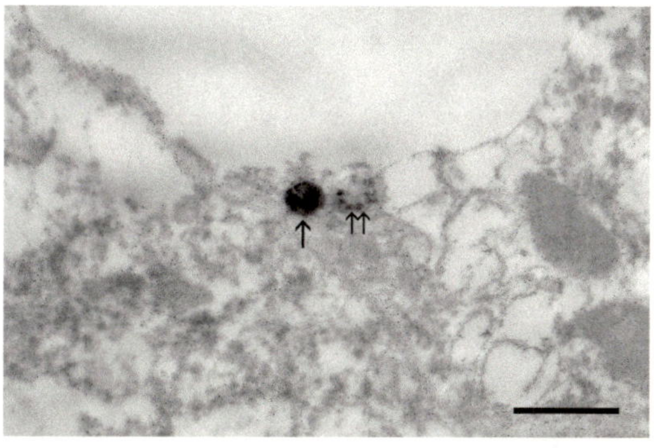

Figure 13. Lungs of the same patient, elementary (double arrow) and reticular (single arrow) bodies of *Chlamydia* detected by electron microscopy (scale 1 μm).

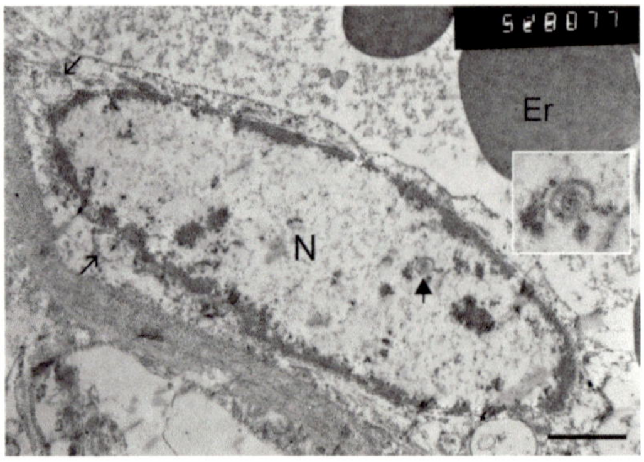

Figure 14. Brain of the same patient, reticular bodies in the cytoplasm and PML inclusion (insertion on the right) in endothelial cell detected by electron microscopy. N, nucleus; Er, erythrocyte (scale 2 μm).

lobar pneumonia are noted. But microscopic picture is quite different: lungs are plethoric; lumen alveoli contain serous exudate (but practically no neutrophils), occasionally erythrocytes; and the most typical and important were hyaline membranes (**Figure 15**). Microthrombosis of arterioles and venules was noted as well (**Figure 16**). Such changes were not typical for lethal outcomes due to former virus types. We can assume that such changes could be explained by cytokine overproduction by damaged macrophages, but such hypothesis needs to be proven by proper methods.

6. Extrapulmonary manifestations with involvement of the brain, meninges, heart (**Figure 17**), vessels, kidneys, liver, and intestine in severe influenza occur rather regularly. Partly, they can be explained by vascular disorders due to not fully clarified "toxic influences," but tropism of certain influenza strains to the brain, intestine, endothelium, and placenta has been either proven or at least suspected. There is also evidence of intrauterine influenza, although usually without severe clinical manifestations. The role of influenza virus in development of malformations has been discussed for a long time but still remains doubtful. The question which

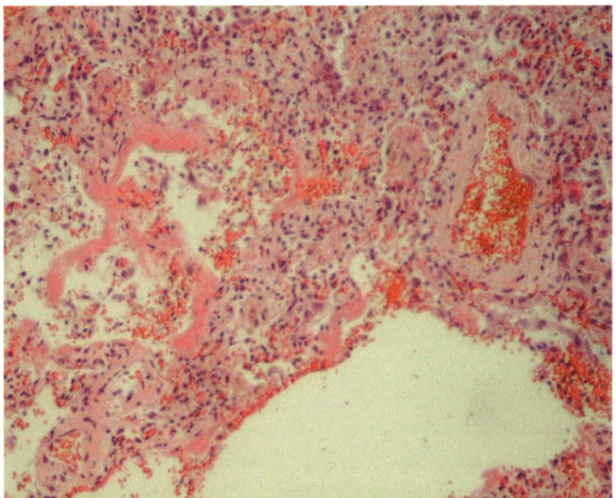

Figure 15. Hyaline membranes in the lung of a patient deceased from influenza a H1N1 swine (H&E, ×600).

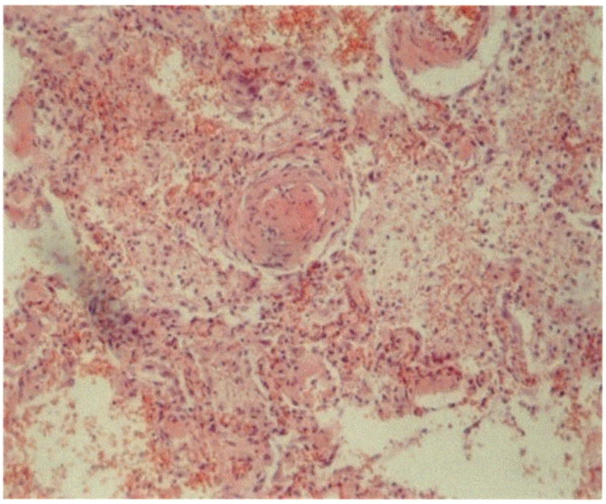

Figure 16. Microthrombosis of the arteriole in the lung of a patient deceased from influenza a H1N1 swine (H&E, ×400).

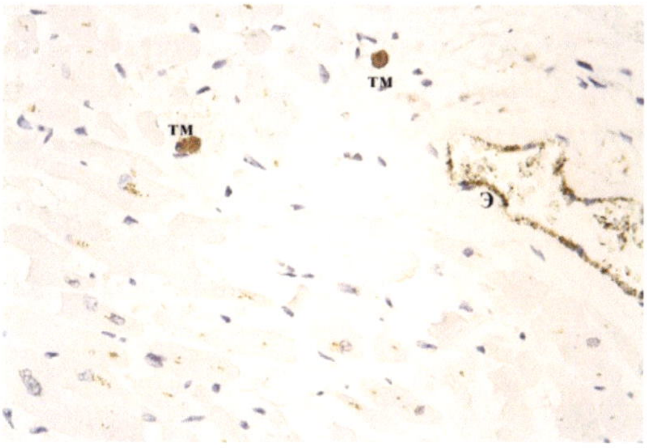

Figure 17. Nuclear protein of influenza a virus in the heart (IHC ×400).

needs further studies is the fact that the antigen of influenza virus is detected outside the respiratory system with the help of IHC or immunofluorescence more frequently than by virus cultivation. The hypothesis of probable appearance of incomplete viral particles or tis-mutants needs to be investigated on clinical material.

7. Immediate death causes in influenza may be quite different. Basing upon our long-term experience, we can distinguish (1) severe respiratory insufficiency due to respiratory distress syndrome, (2) generalized viral infection, (3) secondary bacterial pneumonia, and (4) aggravation of severe somatic diseases. Many aspects of pathogenesis need complex study. It is obvious that such division has extreme clinical importance; unfortunately, we never found similar analysis in the literature.

In experiment the following groups were studied: (1) mice intranasal challenged with influenza viruses A/California/07/09 (H1N1) and A/WSN (H1N1) in saline solution in doses 1 and 10 LD50, and (2) control mice got only saline or were considered as negative control. Virus titer was determined by standard methods.

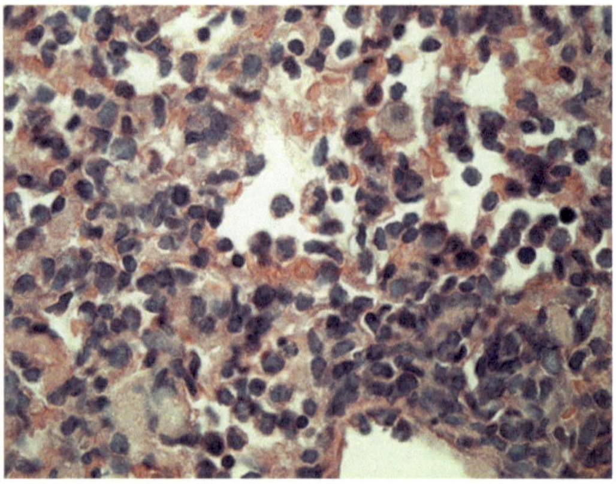

Figure 18. Virus-induced changes in the lung of a mouse on 3D after intranasal challenge with influenza a/California/07/09 (H1N1) (H&E, ×600).

Replication of influenza viruses of both types was maximal on the third day after challenge (California 6.20 ± 0.18; WSN 6.10 ± 0.26) with its gradual decrease on the 7th and 14th day. One has to note that on the 14th day the medium index of replication influenza California virus (1.30 ± 0.30) was more than twice as high as those of A/WSN 0.60 ± 0.22).

The cells of bronchial epithelium, alveolocytes, alveolar macrophages, and endotheliocytes contained viral antigen and underwent changes similar to those described on human autopsy material but expressed moderately (**Figure 18**). Lesions comparable with "diffuse alveolar damage" in men were absent.

Thus, we can resume that the disease caused by different strains of influenza A virus has substantial peculiarities. Histopathological changes are rather typical and allow at least to suspect the etiology of infection, which has to be confirmed by virological methods, RT-PCR nowadays first of all. Lethal outcomes may be related to (1) severe respiratory insufficiency due to respiratory distress syndrome, (2) generalized viral infection, (3) secondary bacterial pneumonia, and (4) aggravation of somatic diseases, ischemic heart disease first of all. Many questions of influenza pathogenesis need to be clarified in complex studies on clinical and experimental material including morphological methods. Among the most important studies which have to be provided, we can mention (1) the exact virus-cell interactions in the target cells and mechanism of cytoproliferative changes; (2) interactions of influenza with other viruses, bacteria, mycoplasma and fungi; (3) the nature of extrapulmonary lesions; and (4) the difference in histopathological picture due to the same virus type in different species.

Author details

Vsevolod A. Zinserling

Address all correspondence to: zinserling@yandex.ru

National Federal Research Center named after V.A. Almazov, Saint-Petersburg University, Clinical Infectious Hospital named after SP Botkin, Saint-Petersburg, Russia

References

[1] Thangavel RR, Bouvier NM. Animal models for influenza virus pathogenesis, transmission, and immunology. Journal of Immunological Methods. Aug 2014;**Apr 4**:60-79. DOI: 10.1016/j.jim.2014.03.023

[2] Kradin RL, editor. Diagnostic Pathology of Infectious Disease 1st ed. Philadelfia: Saunders Elsevier; 2010. ISBN: 978-1-4160-3429-2

[3] Milner DA, editor. Diagnostic pathology. In: Infectious Diseases. 1st ed. Philadelfia: Elsevier; 2015. ISBN: 978-0-323-37677-8

[4] Gill JR, Sheng Z-M, Ely SF, et al. Pulmonary pathologic findings of fatal 2009 pandemic influenza A/H1N1 viral infections. Archives of Pathology & Laboratory Medicine. 2010; **134**:235-243

[5] Mauad T, Hajjar LA, Callegari GD, et al. Lung pathology in fatal novel human influenza A (H1N1) infection. American Journal of Respiratory and Critical Care Medicine. Jan 1, 2010;**181**(1):72-79

[6] Nakajima N, Hata S, Sato Y, et al. The first autopsy case of pandemic influenza (A/H1N1pdm) virus infection in Japan: Detection of a high copy number of the virus in type II alveolar epithelial cells by pathological and virological examination. Japanese Journal of Infectious Diseases. 2010;**63**:67-71

[7] Bhatnagar J, Jones T, Blau DM, et al. Localization of pandemic 2009 H1N1 influenza A virus RNA in lung and lymph nodes of fatal influenza cases by situ hybridization: New insights on virus replication and pathogenesis. Journal of Clinical Virology. 2013;**56**(3):232-237. DOI: 10.1016/j.jcv.11.014

[8] Capelozzi VL, Parra ER, Ximenes M, et al. Pathological and ultrastructural analysis of surgical lung biopsies in patients with swine-origin influenza type A/H1N1 and acute respiratory failure. Clinics. 2010;**65**(12):1229-1237

[9] Merzt D, Geraci J, Wincup J, et al. Pregnancy as a risk factor for severe outcomes from influenza virus infection: A systemic review and meta-analysis of observational studies. Vaccine. 2016;**35**(4):521-528. DOI: 10.1016/j.vaccine.2016.12.012

[10] Zinserling (Tsinzerling) VA. Etiology and Pathologic Anatomy of Acute Respiratory Infections (in Russian). Leningrad: Meditsina; 1977

[11] Zinserling VA. Peculiarities of lesions in viral and mycoplasma infections of respiratory tract. Virchows Archiv. 1972;**356**:259-273

[12] Zinserling VA, Aksenov OA, Melnikova VF, Zinserling VA. Extrapulmonary lesions in influenza. Tohoku Journal of Experimental Medicine. 1983;**140**:259-272

[13] Zinserling VA, Vorobjev SL, Zarubajev VV, et al. Pathogenic aspects of influenza during the epidemics caused by virus H1N1v in 2009-2010 on autopsies. Arkhiv Patologii (Moskwa). 2011;**73**(6):21-25 (in Russian)

[14] Yakovlev AA, Zinserling VA, Esaulenko EV. Lethal outcomes in influenza: Clinic-pathological approach to immediate death causes (in Russian). Journal of Infectologii. 2017;**9**(4):53-59. DOI: 10.22625/2072-6732-2017-9-4-53-58

[15] Zinserling VA, Dedov VA Influenza. In: Hofman P, editor. Infectious Disease and Parasites. Berlin: Springer; 2016. DOI: 10.1007/978-3-319-300009-2

[16] Zinserling VA. Immediate death causes in influenza. Virchows Archiv. 2017;**471**(S.1):s100

Section 3

Prevention of Influenza

Chapter 3

Preventing Zoonotic Influenza

Clement Meseko, Binod Kumar and Melvin Sanicas

Additional information is available at the end of the chapter

http://dx.doi.org/10.5772/intechopen.76966

Abstract

The public health risk of influenza at the human-animal interface is dicey, due in part to continuous evolution of the virus. Influenza virus consist of 7 genera of which only influenza A is at present zoonotic, where subtypes H5, H7 and H9 of avian origin and subtype H1 and H3 of swine origin are important. The most devastating influenza pandemic in history was suspected to have emerged from avian reservoir and manifested in 1918. The first recognized direct human transmission of highly pathogenic avian influenza (HPAI) H5N1 occurred in 1997 in Hong Kong. Subsequently, many cases of varying severity have been described in people who were exposed to poultry. More recently in 2009, triple reassortant influenza A of swine origin (A/H1N1pdm09) caused the first pandemic of the twenty-first century and since 2013, H7N9 though initially benign in birds, caused fatal infection in humans who had contact with poultry. These public health threats from animal influenza virus are aggravated by increase co-mingling in shared human-animal environment. Therefore, the challenge of emerging zoonotic influenza viruses on human host immunity, efficacy of vaccines and antiviral resistance require continuous risk assessment of virological and clinical changes that have impact on control measures including advances in vaccines and chemotherapeutics.

Keywords: influenza viruses, zoonotic transmission, reassortment, immunity and vaccines, antiviral resistance

1. Historical perspective on zoonotic influenza

The family of influenza virus, known as *Orthomyxoviridae*, consists of 7 genera viz.: Influenza A, B, C and D. Others are *Thogotovirus*, *Quaranjavirus* and *Isavirus* which are associated with arthropods and fish [1]. Only 3, influenza A, B and C so far have been described in humans, while only Influenza A is commonly transmitted from animals to human and vice versa [2, 3]. Influenza A virus (IAV) is further divided into subtypes based on the Hemagglutinin surface glycoproteins (HA1-18) and Neuraminidase (NA1-11), HA1-16 and NA1-9 are those that are up till date identified to occur naturally in avian host, mostly waterfowls where they exist in benign form (low pathogenic) [4, 5]. Two additional subtypes (HA 17 and 18, NA 10 and 11) were identified in bats [6]. Genetic mutations and reassortment may occur spontaneously or over a long period in reservoir hosts. These result in the emergence of novel subtypes, reassortants, strains or variants from the Low Pathogenic Avian Influenza (LPAI) precursors. These phenomena that have been described as antigenic shift and drift also contribute to the evolution, adaptation and inter-species transmission of influenza viruses and provide opportunities for gain of function in nature including molecular and or biological properties that may enhance zoonotic transmission. Sometimes a strain may arise in animals with adaptations of fitness to cause fatal infection or increase transmission and potentials to cause pandemics in human population [7, 8].

Aquatic birds are the most important group of animals in the ecology and epidemiology of influenza virus. Almost all naturally circulating subtypes of influenza virus in birds and mammals (including human) can be traced to avian descendants including earlier description in literature by Perroncito in 1878 [4, 9]. The first pandemic of influenza virus that occurred in 1918 (Spanish flu) was caused by an avian influenza virus, as revealed by sero-archeology and molecular characterization [10, 11]. The 1918 influenza pandemic killed over 50 million people and about one third (500 million persons) of the world's population had clinically apparent illnesses. The Case-fatality rate was greater than 2.5% in comparison to less than 0.1% in other influenza pandemics. Nearly half of influenza-related deaths were observed in young adults between the ages of 20–40 years, an indication that the virus was newly introduced possibly from animal reservoir to naive human population [12].

The causative virus of the 1918 pandemic, following human transmission, was concurrently transmitted to pigs in America, Europe and China. This was to play out again in 2009 when A/H1N1pdm09 virus was also transmitted via anthropogenic means to swine. In both scenarios, the causative virus was eventually isolated in pigs [2, 13]. More epidemics and pandemics arising from descendants of the 1918 virus were subsequently recorded in 1957 Asian flu (H2N2), 1968 Hong Kong flu (H3N2) and the more recent H1N1 2009 influenza pandemic that originated in Mexico (Mexican flu). The common precursor of these viruses appeared to be an avian influenza virus that entered the human population directly or indirectly through intermediate hosts probably at some points involving pigs as enunciated by Nelson et al. [14] and in **Figure 1**. Exceptionally, the 1918 pandemic virus appeared to have been wholly derived from avian-like influenza virus from an unknown source [15]. Thus zoonotic influenza transmission seems to be the foundation of influenza virus infection in human including previous pandemics, contemporary and more recent transmissions and fatal human infections caused by avian H5, H7 and H9 in many countries [16, 17].

In the last 100 years, influenza virus in human are generally manifested as seasonal, zoonotic and pandemic with clinico-pathological manifestation that vary from mild, severe to fatal. However, the most threatening influenza infections are those caused by zoonotic and/or pandemic strains following their introduction usually from animal reservoir into human population that has little or no pre-existing specific or cross protective immunity [18]. The burden of

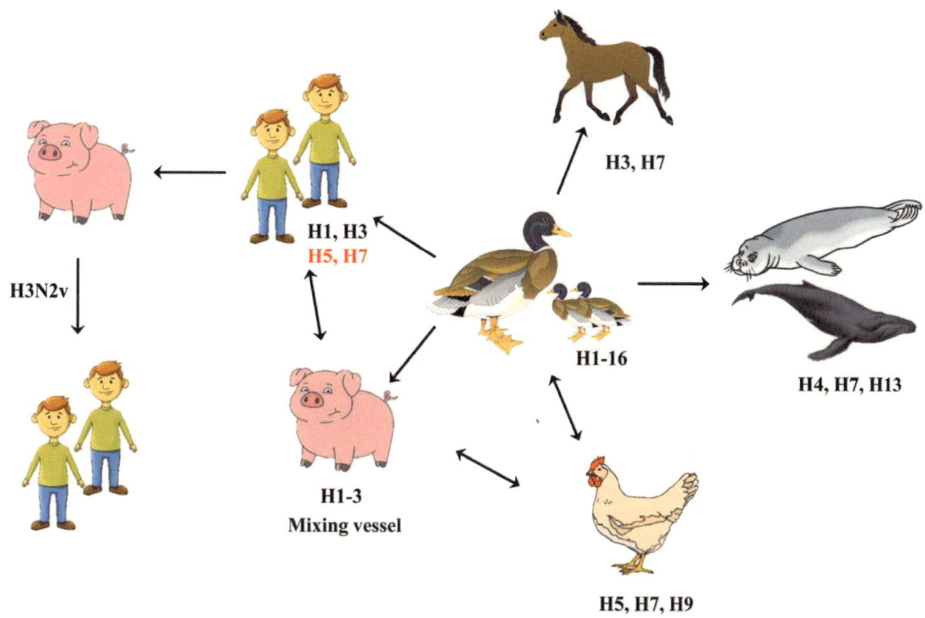

Figure 1. Illustration of cross-species transmission of avian, swine and human influenza viruses. Waterfowls as natural reservoirs, pigs serve as 'mixing vessels', viruses from humans seed pH1N1 in swine populations, reassortment between pH1N1 viruses and co-circulating triple reassortant H3N2 viruses in pigs generate novel reassortant H3N2v.

zoonotic and potentially pandemic influenza A virus infections has therefore attracted global concern since the identification of avian and swine influenza viruses that can (with or without biological or molecular adaptations) be transmitted directly, and cause severe disease in humans and other mammals. This was notable with the advent of A/Goose/Guangdong/96 lineage of H5N1, which had infected 860 people and killed 454 (52% case-fatality rate) up till December 2017 [19]. Continuous circulation of H5N1 in birds and zoonotic transmission to human may cause influenza virus to acquire adaptive genetic features for efficient human to human transmission through mutations (insertions/deletions), reassortment or emergence of immune or antiviral resistant strains. Those may likely be precursors of emerging influenza virus with pandemic potential. Global surveillance for influenza diversity in animals and human may therefore greatly improve our ability for early detection, to identify and anticipate which strains are more likely to evolve and be better prepared [18].

2. Human infections with avian influenza virus

The first human transmission of Highly Pathogenic Avian Influenza (HPAI) subtype H5N1 occurred in 1997 in Hong Kong. It became a global public health concern, knowing that pandemic influenza viruses in the past originated from animals [20]. The H5N1 was thus considered a potential pandemic threat [21]. The HPAI H5N1 lineage (A/Goose/Guangdong/1/96) was initially isolated from a goose farm in Guangdong Province, China in 1996. In the following year, outbreaks of highly pathogenic H5N1 were reported in poultry at farms and live bird markets in Hong Kong. Subsequently, contact with poultry and exposure to infected live and/or dead birds became the medium for human exposure and in Hong Kong there were altogether, 18 cases (6 fatal) reported in the first known instance of human infection with this virus [22].

Early symptoms of influenza H5N1 virus usually develop 2 to 4 days after exposure to sick poultry and most patients infected with influenza H5N1 virus presents symptoms of fever, cough, shortness of breath and radiological evidence of pneumonia [21]. The number of human H5N1 cases reported globally was heightened in 2003 and since then, the virus has maintained a steady infection, morbidity and mortality at the animal-human interface. Those primarily at risk are cohorts of poultry farmers, handlers and operators in live bird markets and their immediate family members or contact. Though human to human transmission of H5N1 is not yet efficient, evolving nature of influenza virus in the environment is a reminder of the risk of emergence of a strain adapted for that possibility.

The HPAI (H5, H7) viruses circulating in terrestrial poultry (Chicken and turkeys) and are transmitted to human, normally emerge from the low pathogenic precursors in waterfowls. This arises by mutations in the gene and occurrence of multiple basic amino acids in the connecting peptide between the HA1 and HA2 domains of the HA0 precursor protein [23]. Trypsin-like proteases found in the respiratory and gastrointestinal tracts may be responsible for this limited enzymatic cleavage hence pathology are usually restricted to these systems. However, when multiple basic amino acids are introduced by insertion or deletion in the HA cleavage site, the HA0 precursor becomes cleavable by a wide range of ubiquitous proteases found in many host tissues [24]. Consequently, the virus is able to replicate in almost all the tissues/organs beside the respiratory and gastrointestinal tracts such as brain (nervous) and the cardiovascular (hematopoietic) system, resulting in fulminant and disseminated disease with high mortality index particularly in turkey and chicken [25].

In a peculiar incident, in February and March 2013, three patients were hospitalized with severe lower respiratory tract disease of unknown cause in China. The causative virus was later identified as novel avian-origin reassortant influenza A (H7N9), and phylogenetic analysis of all genes of the isolate showed that each gene segment was of avian origin [17]. The HA cleavage site possessed only a single basic amino acid R (arginine) as against polybasic, indicating tendency to be of low pathogenicity in poultry. On the contrary, cases in human host were severe, with patients developing severe pneumonia, acute respiratory distress, and eventually death. All the three patients had pre-existing medical conditions, but more importantly two of them had a history of direct contact with poultry [17]. The switch in virulence and pathogenicity were associated with certain mutations in the reassorted virus that may have contributed to severity of human infection and death. Similarly, waves of H5N8 outbreaks, first detected in domestic birds in China in 2010, which later spread from 2014 through 2016 in Europe and North America was heighten in the winter of 2016 and affected a wide range of domestic and wild birds but no human infection was recorded. Experimental studies even showed low virulence in ferret hence risks to human were considered low [26], even though the contemporary HPAI viruses of subtypes H5N2, H5N5, H5N6 and H5N8, all contain genes from 1997 A/Goose/Guangdong H5N1 lineage with acquired internal genes from LPAIs. Interestingly, the H5N8 (clade 2.3.4.4) though virulent in poultry has remained of low susceptibility in human, but another newly emerged H5N6 first identified in a peafowl arising from reassortment of H5 clade 2.3.4.4 has shown virulence in human and has killed 7 people among 17 that were infected since 2016 [27]. Repeated cases in human have raised concerns that subtype H5N6 virus also has the potential for crossover human infection which if sustained, may also be a candidate for influenza pandemic [28]. The notification of the first human case of novel subtype H7N4 to the Centre for Health Protection in Hong Kong on the 14th of February 2018 is a reminder that avian influenza is continually evolving bird-human transmission [29]. This H7N4 event and previous H7N9 detection first in human before cases in poultry were noticed also shows that humans are fast becoming sentinel for influenza surveillance at the human-animal interface.

3. The pandemic H1N1pdm09, zoonosis and reverse zoonosis

Triple reassortant influenza A/H1N1pdm09 originating in swine caused the 1st pandemic of the twenty-first century in 2009. This was at the time of HPAI H5N1 epizootics in Asia, Europe and Africa. The strain and the region thought to be probable epicenter of future pandemic was H5N1 and Asia. The severity and spread of HPAI H5N1 in poultry and subsequent transmission to human, lent credence to scientific speculations that the zoonotic virus might have been a pandemic strain. Unpredictably, while attention was on HPAI H5N1, a pandemic H1N1 influenza virus emerged in Mexico, although the virus was believed to have been circulating in pigs many years before its first detection in human [16, 30]. The 2009 influenza pandemic spread to more than 214 countries and an estimated 151,700–575,400 respiratory and cardiovascular deaths were associated with the infection worldwide [31]. Lessons learnt include the realization that a zoonotic and pandemic virus may emerge from an animal reservoir in an unexpected location and spread rapidly throughout the world within a short time [32]. Also important is the realization that that the 2009 H1N1 pandemic virus was subsequently transmitted from human to pigs in a phenomenon that has been variously described as reverse zoonosis reported in more than 20 countries in America, Europe, Asia and Africa. Interestingly, the swine influenza sequence data available in public gene bank showed that humans transmit far more influenza A virus to swine than pigs have ever transmitted to humans, at least in terms of viruses that are transmitted onward in the new host as against dead end or accidental hosts [14]. The implication is that endemic human-like influenza virus that is enzootic in pigs will continuously pose public health risk in the generation of Influenza variants (combination of human and swine influenza viruses). This has also been reported to cause human infections in people exposed to pigs especially in America [14].

Virus strains or variants resulting from reassortment of swine influenza A(H3N2) and influenza A/H1N1pdm09 and similar viruses have been detected in swine in many countries. It is therefore of concern that emerging influenza variants could efficiently be transmitted among humans. Over 300 human cases of A(H3N2)v have been described between 2011 and 2012 in the United State alone beside clusters of human-human transmission further demonstrating that variant influenza viruses also pose a public health threat at the human-animal interface. Animals and humans may infect each other in intensive farms, abattoirs and agricultural fairs when in close proximity [33, 34]. Our ability to predict and prevent outbreaks of zoonotic pathogens like influenza therefore requires an understanding of their ecology and evolution in reservoir hosts [35]. This is important because Influenza A viruses from animals including reassortant, novel and variants are considered of significant threat in the emergence of the next pandemic due to the abundance of permanent animal reservoirs harboring viruses that are now frequently spilling over into human.

4. Mutation, reassortment and variants influenza virus

Over the past 100 years, the IAVs have caused several pandemics including the one that has been described as "the greatest medical holocaust in history" [36]. Mutation and reassortment are two well established factors that have contributed in zoonotic influenza viruses gaining the ability to adapt to humans, leading to pandemics and thereafter sustained human-to-human transmissions. The accumulation of mutations and genome reassortments have been the driving force for most of the IAV adaptability in humans as the IAV RNA genome replication lacks the exonuclease proofreading capability, thus giving rise to high nucleotide mutation rates [37]. Antigenic drift and shift are the two major phenomena in influenza viruses that lead to antigenically variant influenza viruses [1, 38, 39]. The antigenic drift refers to point mutations in the HA and/or NA while the antigenic shift leads to the formation of a new virus subtype with a novel combination of HA and NA from different subtypes. While the antigenic drift is responsible for yearly epidemics, the antigenic shift has been responsible for some of the devastating pandemics in influenza history claiming many lives, including the 1918-Spanish flu. A list of zoonotic influenza outbreaks have been summarized in **Table 1**.

The human influenza viruses have limited subtypes of HA and NA (H1, H2, H3 and N1, N2) whereas the avian influenza viruses infecting the poultry may harbor almost all the subtypes of HA and NA [40], thus giving rise to multiple recombination of HA and NA in avian species. Since 1996, the HPAI-H5N1virus have claimed several lives resulting in high mortality rate while the recently identified LPAI-H7N9 in East China region had a mortality rate of 40% [41]. The H7N9 virus isolates have the capability of binding to both avian and human influenza virus receptors due to presence of a leucine at amino acid position 217 [42]. A relatively limited number of mutations in the zoonotic IAV genome can lead to production of new viral progenies with capability of efficient transmission among mammals and studies have also demonstrated that amino acid substitutions in the HA protein can change the preference of binding receptors of influenza viruses. For example, the G186 V mutation in HA protein of H7N9 virus has been identified as the potential adaptation of the virus to human-type receptors [43]. A recent study conducted on a non-laboratory-adapted virus A/Vietnam/1203/2004 (H5N1) with an HA2-K58I point mutation (K to I at position 58) showed that a decrease in the HA activation pH (pH 5.5) influenced the viral properties as compared to the wild type virus (HA activation pH 6.0) in mammalian hosts [44]. The mutation increased the viral load in ferret's nasal cavity while it reduced the viral load in lungs thus supporting the fact that a single mutation could lead to an increased viral growth in mammalian upper respiratory tract [44].

Year (Country)	Influenza subtype	Confirmed cases	Adaptation in segment
1997/2003-present (Asia, Europe and Africa)	H5N1	660	N224 K (HA)
			N158D (HA)
			T160A (HA)
			E627K (PB2)
2003 (USA)	H7N2	1	Not determined
2003 (Hong Kong)	H9N2	1	Q226L (HA)
			G228S (HA)
			T212A (HA)
2003 (The Netherlands)	H7N7	89	E627K (PB2)
2004 (Egypt)	H10N7	2	Not determined
2004 (Canada)	H7N3	2	Not determined
2007 (UK)	H7N2	4	Not determined
2008–2009 (Hong Kong)	H9N2	2	Not determined
2012 (Mexico)	H7N3	2	Not determined
2013 (China)	H10N8	3	Not determined
2013 (China, Taiwan, Hong Kong)	H7N9	137	Q226L (HA)
			E627K (PB2)
2013 (Taiwan)	H6N1	1	P186L (HA)
Since 2014 (China)	H5N6	16	G540A (NS)
2018 (China)	H7N4	1	Not determined

Table 1. Zoonotic influenza A viruses and identified adaptations (reviewed in [53] with modification).

Several studies in ferrets have shown that the viruses such as H5N1 [45], H7N9 [46] and H7N1 [47] could transmit through respiratory droplets after acquiring mutations in their genomes. Another study on A/Anhui/1/13 (H7N9) virus showed that substitutions at G219S and K58I resulted in high affinity for α2,6-linked sialic acid receptor and acid and temperature stability [48]. The increased polymerase activity due to mutation in the viral PB2 has also been linked to enhanced viral replication. The PB2 subunit from all avian viruses generally contains polymerases with glutamic acid at amino acid position 627 (E627) while the PB2 from human viral isolates almost exclusively have lysine at 627 (K627). Mehle et al. have shown that E627K mutation of PB2 conferred a high level of polymerase activity in human and porcine cells thus increasing the viral replication [49]. Another study showed that a basic amino acid at position 591 of the PB2 subunit compensated for the lack of PB2-627 K in HPAI-H5N1 and pandemic H1N1viruses markedly increased the replication of these viruses in mammalian species [50]. The PB2 gene mutation in duck H7N9 also enhanced the polymerase activity and thus viral replication in human cells [51]. The H1N1 influenza virus that caused the 1918 pandemic and the H5N1 avian influenza virus isolated in 1997 (Hong Kong) both harbors the N66S mutation in PB1-F2 which drastically enhanced the pathogenicity of these viruses [52].

Genetic reassortment in influenza viruses is yet another vital event that leads to sudden outbreaks of influenza. Influenza viruses have a segmented genome and thus, simultaneous infection with other IAVs results in reassortment event leading to formation of new viral progenies containing gene segments of mixed parental origin. Several pandemics have emerged in the past [54] and appears to be more frequent now than previously thought [55]. The reassortment event can be a result of errors during the replication of viral RNA polymerase, the host environment, the immune or evolutionary pressure [56]. The pandemics of 1957 and 1968 were caused by reassortant viral strains [57]. The HA, NA, and PB1 genes of the H2N2 1957 pandemic strain and the HA and PB1 fragments of the H3N2 1968 pandemic strain were both derived from avian influenza virus strains [57]. The HPAI subtype H5N1 isolated from geese in Guangdong province in 1996 evolved to produce H5N8 clades 2.3.4.4 Gs/GD HPAIV. A recent study on the evolution and pathogenicity of H5N2 avian influenza viruses isolated in H5N1 endemic areas in China revealed that these viral isolates were derived from reassortment events in which few isolates had the HA and NS derived from H5N1 while few had the HA derived from endemic H9N2 viruses [58]. A similar study from South Korea reported the emergence of novel reassortant H5N8 viruses in 2014 in ducks raised in breeder farms [59]. Since its first appearance, lineage of the HPAI H5N1 continues to circulate with lots of diversification of the HA gene into multiple genetic clades. The H5 clade 2.3.4.4 of the H5N8 subtype was subsequently detected in several countries of Europe by the end of 2014 and in summer of 2016, it was detected again in wild aquatic birds sampled in western Siberia [60]. A recent study has also shown that the reassortment event between the Gs/GD lineage H5N8 virus and North American origin viruses further resulted in the emergence of H5N1 and H5N2 viruses in the US [61].

Experimental observations have further revealed that reassortment between zoonotic and seasonal IAVs can result in production of airborne-transmissible viruses in mammals [62–65]. A study showed that a reassortant virus, comprising of the H5 hemagglutinin having 4 mutations from H5N1 avian virus and remaining seven segments from the 2009 pandemic H1N1 virus lead to reassortant H5 HA/H1N1 virus that gained the capacity of droplet transmission in ferret model [62]. Another experiment further showed that the avian H5N1 subtype viruses do have the potential to attain mammalian transmissibility by genetic reassortment [63]. The authors utilized reverse genetics to create several reassortant viruses between duck H5N1 (HA gene) and human-infective H1N1 virus to show that the new reassortant viruses could efficiently infect and sustained droplet transmission in guinea pigs without mortality [63]. Similar study reported that the avian-human H9N2 reassortant virus harboring the surface proteins of avian H9N2 in a human H3N2 backbone gained the ability of transmission through the respiratory droplets and caused clinical infection in ferrets similar to human influenza infections [64]. A recent study performed in a novel transfection-based inoculation system generated a reassortant H9N1 virus by transfecting the plasmids containing genes from H9N2 virus and pandemic H1N1 (pH1N1) virus into HEK 293 T cells. The resulting transfections gave rise to two reassortant viruses (H9N1) that had the capability of droplet-transmissibility [65].

According to the Centers for Disease Control and Prevention (CDC), when an influenza virus that normally circulates in swine (not in humans) is detected in humans, it is referred to as variant influenza viruses. The human infections with H1N1, H3N2 and H1N2 variant viruses have been reported from United States [13, 65]. Although the variant influenza viruses rarely show sustained human-to-human transmission, yet there have been few strains that overcame this barrier. All the cases reported in US were of swine origin rather than avian origin. In 2009, triple reassortant variant influenza virus was detected throughout the world and caused the first pandemic of twenty-first century. This variant virus had genes from avian, human, and swine influenza viruses claiming more than 12,500 lives in the US alone and about 575,400 globally [31, 66]. Later H3N2 variant viruses which had similarity with triple-reassortant viruses were detected in US swine but had acquired the matrix gene from highly transmissible influenza A H1N1-2009 viruses which contributed in efficiency of transmission of the variant virus [67]. A recent study has also identified two distinct variants of H3N2 influenza virus that grows in cell culture [68]. Both the variants differed in just one single mutation at amino acid 151 of NA. The D151 viral variant could efficiently grow in cell culture while the G151 viral variant showed extremely poor growth in cell culture system [68]. More in-depth studies are still needed to better understand the viral properties of variant influenza viruses as they continue to pose threat to human lives.

5. Immunity and challenges of vaccination

The isolation of influenza A/H1N1 in 1933 quickly ushered the development of the first generation of live-attenuated influenza vaccines (LAIV). The initially developed inactivated influenza vaccine (IIV) only targeted a single influenza strain (influenza A). Then, in 1942, a vaccine targeting both influenza A and B viruses were produced soon after the discovery of influenza B. Subsequently, scientists discovered that influenza viruses mutated, leading to antigenic changes (antigenic drift and antigenic shift). Since 1973, the World Health Organization (WHO) has been providing yearly recommendations for the composition of the influenza vaccine, based on results of the virological surveillance conducted by the WHO's Global Influenza Surveillance and Response System (GISRS). Later in 1978, the trivalent influenza vaccine was developed that included two influenza A strains and one influenza B strain. Currently, two influenza B lineages are circulating (Yamagata and Victoria) therefore, since 2013, the WHO recommendations suggested a second B strain to be added to make a quadrivalent influenza vaccine (QIV) [69]. Influenza vaccines protect against infection and can reduce illness and severity of infection especially in groups at risk for flu complications such as children, the elderly, pregnant women, and individuals with underlying medical conditions like asthma, HIV/AIDS, and chronic heart or lung diseases [70]. Frequent influenza infections at the human-animal interface may also warrant occupational vaccination for veterinarians, researchers, health care providers, farmers and animal traders who are more likely to be exposed to zoonotic influenza virus [71].

For over half a century now, WHO has been collaborating with scientists, epidemiologists, and policymakers to create an integrated approach to manufacture, test, and approve influenza vaccine research and development efforts, including their proper use and efficient distribution. Since the virus mutates frequently, WHO, GISRS network and collaborating centers predict the strains that are expected to circulate in the following season because of the time required to manufacture vaccines. This happens twice a year, one for the northern hemisphere and another for the southern hemisphere [70]. But the virus can mutate during the time it takes to develop the vaccine, resulting in a mismatch between circulating virus and the vaccine.

Although the effectiveness of the flu vaccine varies from year to year depending mainly on the match of the strain in the vaccine and the circulating strain, most provide modest to high protection against influenza [72]. The US-CDC has reported that flu vaccination reduces medical visits, flu illness, hospitalizations, and deaths [73]. Vaccination is still the most efficient way to prevent infection and severe outcomes caused by influenza viruses.

The WHO and CDC recommend yearly vaccination for nearly everyone over 6 months of age, especially those at higher risk of influenza complications and mortality [70, 73]. The European Centre for Disease Prevention and Control (ECDC) also recommends yearly vaccination of high risk groups: older adults and all persons (over 6 months of age) with chronic medical conditions including those with diseases of the respiratory system (e.g. asthma), cardiovascular system (e.g. coronary artery disease), endocrine system (e.g. diabetes), hepatic system (e.g. liver cirrhosis), renal system (e.g. chronic renal failure), neurological/neuromuscular conditions (e.g. parkinsonism), any condition compromising respiratory functions e.g. morbid obesity (BMI > 40), physical handicap in children and adults, and immunosuppression due to disease or treatment including due to hematological conditions and HIV infection [74].

Currently licensed flu vaccines include inactivated influenza vaccine (IIV), live attenuated influenza vaccine (LAIV), and recombinant HA vaccines [75]. These vaccines are either trivalent or quadrivalent with components representing influenza A and B viruses predicted to circulate in the next influenza season. The IIV is either a split virion or subunit vaccine containing 15 μg of each purified HA protein administered intramuscularly, or 9 μg of each purified HA protein administered intradermally [75]. A higher dose version with 60 μg of each HA antigen is available for older adults aged 65 years and above. The IIV induces a strain-specific serum IgG antibody response. A vaccine with an oil-in-water adjuvant MF59 also enhances the immunogenicity of IIV in the elderly [76].

The LAIV contains live viruses with temperature-sensitive and attenuating mutations [77] and is a combination of the same four strains as the QIV. The LAIV is administered intranasally as a spray. The mutations in the LAIV strains allow the viruses to replicate at the cooler temperature of the nasal cavity but prohibit replication at the temperature of the lower respiratory tract. The LAIV results in the production of strain-specific serum IgG as well as mucosal IgA and T cell responses [77]. The recombinant HA vaccine with HA proteins expressed in insect cells from baculovirus vectors is currently licensed only for adults aged 18 to 49 years and are recommended for individuals who are allergic to eggs [75]. The manufacturing process for the recombinant HA vaccine is shorter than the IIV and LAIV, which would be important in case of a pandemic. The 2009 pandemic showed the challenges in production and distribution of vaccines against a newly emerged virus within a short timeframe given the production timeline for both IIV and LAIV [78]. Production of IIV and LAIV require the use of embryonated eggs. Disadvantages for egg-based flu vaccine production include being contraindicated in people with severe allergies to eggs, and in the event of a pandemic where the virus is pathogenic to poultry, embryonated eggs may be in short supply [69]. Currently, licensed influenza vaccines focus on the production of antibodies against the viral HA protein, which binds host receptors to mediate viral entry. Strain-specific antibodies produced against the HA neutralize the virus and prevent infection. However, the HA is under positive selection for antigenic escape from neutralization by pre-existing antibodies [70].

Vaccine-induced HAI antibody titer is currently accepted as the correlate of protection against influenza. An HAI titer of ≥1:40 in healthy adults is the titer at which approximately 50% of individuals are protected from infection. However, some studies have indicated that a higher HAI titer may be required in children and that T cells may be a better indicator for protection in the elderly [79, 80]. Also, serum HAI antibody titer is not a reliable correlate of protection for seasonal and pandemic LAIV vaccines. LAIV has been shown to be effective in the absence of a robust serum antibody response [77]. The HAI antibody titer also fails to take into account other aspects of immune memory against the virus, including the contribution of non-neutralizing antibodies and T cell responses to protection. The immune response to influenza is complicated, and there could be several correlates of protection apart from HAI antibodies. A more comprehensive immunological analysis and an integrative genomic analysis of the human immune response [81] using the different influenza vaccines could further define other correlates of protection to better interpret influenza vaccine efficacy [82].

Influenza A viruses (IAVs) infects human, swine, and domestic poultry; therefore; interspecies and intercontinental spread make IAV more complicated. Vaccination of domestic poultry (including chicken and turkey) is common against the HPAI, H5/H7 LPAI, and H9N2 LPAI worldwide. In the past, emergency vaccination against HPAI to control epizootics has occurred. Areas include Mexico (H5N1, 1995), Pakistan (H7N3, 1995–2004), Asia/Africa/ Europe (H5N1, 1996–continuing), and North Korea (H7N7, 2005) to aid in stamping out programmes [83]. Poultry vaccines are manufactured inexpensively and are not filtered and purified like human vaccines and usually contain a whole virus, and not just HA antigen. Mineral oil, which induces a strong immune reaction and causes inflammation and abscesses, is added as an adjuvant to poultry vaccines.

Usage of vaccine to control swine influenza virus (SIV) varies by countries; some countries use vaccination strategies, while others do not. For examples, SIV vaccination is conducted extensively in Europe and North America. In Korea, on the other hand, vaccines for SIV control are rarely used despite availability in the market. Because of the genetic diversity of circulating SIV strains, most commercial vaccines consist of multiple strains of subtype H1N1, H1N2, and H3N2. Nevertheless, the rapid evolution of circulating viruses could surpass the updates of commercial vaccines. Combining the herd-specific autogenous vaccine with other commercialized vaccines occurs in some countries; about 20% of pig farms in the United States used autogenous vaccines in 2006. However, compared to avian influenza viruses, vaccines against SIVs have not been used extensively by swine veterinarians in many countries because other major pathogens including the porcine reproductive syndrome virus and porcine circovirus are considered more important [83]. Nevertheless, successful application of influenza vaccines in animals may contribute in reducing zoonotic transmission.

6. Antiviral resistance mutants

Antiviral resistance in influenza viruses is a global concern and the number of resistant mutants is increasing year after year. The antiviral drugs have been formulated mainly against the M2 ion channel (amantadine and rimantadine) and the neuraminidase proteins (oseltamivir and zanamivir) of influenza viruses. These FDA approved drugs are currently used for prophylaxis and treatment of influenza A infections and are effective against the HPAI H5N1 viruses [84]. The effectiveness of these drugs ranges from 80 to 90% if the treatment had begun within 48 hours of infection [85]. The antiviral resistance in influenza may develop during disease treatment and occasionally spreads widely to replace the susceptible strains in the absence of drug pressure. An example of this event is the global spread of adamantane-resistant H3N2 viruses in the year 2003, oseltamivir-resistant seasonal H1N1 viruses since 2007 and more recently the adamantane-resistant pandemic A (H1N1) viruses in 2009. Such events show the highly unpredictable nature of influenza viruses and increase the challenge of its management. Sometimes a single reassortment event or mutations leads to emergence of variant influenza viruses such as the pandemic 2009 or seasonal A (H1N1) viruses that becomes completely unresponsive to most antiviral drugs. The amantadine resistance was soon observed after the discovery of the drug in early 1960s and studies subsequently reported that a single point mutation in the M2 protein lead to the emergence of high-level resistant mutant viruses showing resistance to both amantadine and rimantadine [86]. Other studies also suggested that resistance to M2 blockers (amantadine/rimantadine) can be achieved by only a few substitutions in the codon L26, L27, A30, A31 and G34 of the M2 gene [87] and these mutants retain the virulence and are transmissible between humans [88]. A study showed that adamantane resistance emerged in about 30% of patients post few days of treatment [89]. Another study has shown the synergistic antiviral effects of amantadine-oseltamivir combination chemotherapy [90]. The adamantanes were very effective for almost 4 decades after which the frequency of adamantine resistance among influenza A H3N2 viruses started to increase. The global resistance among H3N2 virus was as low as 0.8% between the periods 1991 to 1995. The adamantine resistance has now been reported for human H1N1, H3N2 and H5N1 avian influenza viruses. The frequency of resistance further increased to 28% during 2004–2005 and to 72% in 2005–2006 for H1N1 variant viruses [1]. The US reported around 92% resistance among H3N2 viruses by the year 2005. A recent study based on the frequency and distribution of M2 gene mutations in influenza virus variants that circulated between 1902 and 2013 showed that 45.2% of all resistant influenza A viruses (H1-H17) circulating globally had S31 N mutations [91].

Similarly the NA mutations causing resistance to neuraminidase inhibitors (NAI) has lots of variations. The most common mutation observed is the H275Y that confers high resistance to oseltamivir [92]. A study showed that the amino acid changes at residue 223 (I → R/V) conferred reduced inhibition to oseltamivir and zanamivir [93]. The N2 subtype has been associated with oseltamivir resistance due to mutation at E119V and R292K. The R292K has also been linked to zanamivir resistance [94]. Studies have demonstrated that the most frequent mutation conferring the oseltamivir resistance in NA of the H1N1 and H5N1 subtypes was H274Y, while the E119V and R292K mutations were more common among the H3N2 and H7N9 subtypes [95]. Another study showed that R292K mutation in NA protein in the H7N9 virus strains were detected in patients after drug treatment. This substitution promoted resistance against oseltamivir [96]. Similarly oseltamivir resistance was associated with the H274Y NA mutation in H5N1 influenza viruses detected in patients during treatment or prophylaxis [97]. Few other studies have reported that the Egyptian H5N1avian influenza isolates from humans had N294S NA mutation [98]. Boltz et al. reported that H5N1 viruses of clade 2.3.2 isolated from the Republic of Laos in 2006–2008 had V116A, I222L, and S246 N mutations in NA [99]. The ongoing concerns about influenza A viruses and increasing antiviral resistance needs immediate attention, better antiviral surveillance for better management and control of future influenza pandemics.

7. Infection control, advances in vaccines and therapeutics

Generally, people infected with the flu are advised to stay home and rest, both to recover and to avoid infecting others. In severe cases, or for individuals at high risk of complications, physicians may prescribe antiviral medication. The antiviral drugs currently available against influenza viruses are adamantane derivatives (amantadine and rimantadine) and neuraminidase (NA) inhibitors (zanamivir, oseltamivir and peramivir). A viral infection can be inhibited at several crucial steps, such as entry, signaling, assembly, and egress [1].

Oseltamivir, works by blocking neuraminidase that enables newly made influenza virus to escape from an infected cell. Zanamivir (inhaled), peramivir (intravenous), and inavir (inhaled) operate in a similar way. Baloxavir, discovered in Osaka, received preliminary approval in Japan in January 2018 and will be filed for regulatory review in the US and Europe thereafter. Baloxavir requires a single dose, unlike oseltamivir which is taken twice a day for 5 days [100].

Efforts to improve currently available vaccines have been explored over the last 2 decades such as: increasing the antigen dose, intradermal route of administration to activate other arms of the immune system, and adding immunostimulating compounds such as adjuvants [78]. The main areas of research and development in flu vaccines involve:

1. Creation of vaccines with protective immunity lasting more than one season,
2. Shortening of the production time to allow a virological assessment nearer the upcoming influenza season. Cell-culture-based vaccines (e.g., Optaflu, Flucelvax, Preflucel, and Celvapan) are also being used to overcome this issue [101].

3. Development of a universal vaccine that protects against influenza regardless of what influenza viruses are circulating. These includes vaccine targeting the HA stalk domain [102, 103], and the use of influenza-virus-like particles as vaccines [104].

In addition to antiviral drugs and vaccines, several novel therapeutic alternatives may prove to be beneficial in the near future. The long-acting inhaled neuraminidase inhibitor CS-8958 (also known as R-118958) has shown promising results in murine models of influenza treatment while a polymerase inhibitor, T-705 (Toyama Chemical), that inhibits viral RNA polymerase has been found to be effective against all three influenza virus types (A, B and C) and to some extent against other RNA viruses, including hemorrhagic fever viruses. The drug, DAS181, a fusion construct that includes the sialidase from *Actinomyces viscosus*, affects the viral attachment process during the early stages of influenza replication. Another study demonstrated the antiviral properties of chlorogenic acid (CHA) and its inhibitory effect on A/PuertoRico/8/1934 (H1N1) and oseltamivir-resistant strains in the late stage of the infectious cycle. Other novel antiviral drugs under clinical development include AVI-7100, a 20-mer phosphorodiamidate morpholino oligomer (PMO) IV formulation that hinders translation and splicing of mRNA from the matrix gene. EV-077, a dual thromboxane receptor antagonist and thromboxane synthase inhibitor, prevents virus replication by inhibiting prostanoids associated with influenza infections. Aureonitol, a compound obtained from fungi, has shown inhibitory effects against both influenza A and B virus replication by impairing virus adsorption. Monoclonal antibodies, CR6261 and CR8020, bind to the conserved stalk region of HA and inhibit the entry and fusion stages. A broad spectrum human monoclonal antibody (mAb- MEDI8852), which unlike other stem-reactive antibodies, used a rare heavy chain VH (VH6-1) gene, was found to be effective in mice and ferrets and better than oseltamivir [1]. These novel approaches will potentially become effective tools for managing seasonal, zoonotic and pandemic influenza virus infections.

8. Conclusions

Influenza viruses have a silent reservoir in the aquatic avian species and continuously pose threat to human population. The avian, swine and other zoonotic influenza infections may range from a mild upper respiratory tract infection to a more severe pneumonia, acute respiratory distress syndrome and even death. Humans can be infected with a wide range of avian [subtypes A(H5N1), A(H7N9), and A(H9N2)] and swine [subtypes A(H1N1), A(H1N2) and A(H3N2)] influenza viruses. Although sustained human to human transmission is lacking, these viruses can be transmitted when there is a direct contact with infected animals or contaminated environments. The virus shows a tremendous potential to mutate, re-assort and give rise novel variants to evade host immunity and vaccination strategies. The emergence of antiviral mutants has further worsened the worldwide control measures. Although management of influenza has been a challenging task owing to its large reservoir and ability to mutate rapidly, the disease can be controlled in the animal source to decrease the risk to human population. With advancements in modern diagnostic methods, vaccination and antiviral strategies, the annual epidemics and occasional pandemics can be managed efficiently.

9. Future perspectives

The public health threats from influenza viruses have always been a global concern. They are not only responsible for annual epidemics throughout the world, but also affect quality of life and have negative impacts on the economy due to frequent school and work place absenteeism. The frequencies of influenza infections have further increased due to co-mingling in shared human-animal environment. The virus is known to acquire antigenic shift and drifts and thus pose challenges in control measures and management. Advancements in vaccination strategies, discovery of novel drugs and antiviral therapeutics along with development of a universal influenza vaccine are promising approaches toward the management of future epidemics and pandemics.

Disclosure of potential conflicts of interest

All authors declared that they have no conflict of interest (financial or non-financial).

Abbreviations

CDC	centers for disease control and prevention
ECDC	European Centre for Disease Prevention and Control
FDA	Food and Drug Administration
GISRS	global influenza surveillance and response system
HA	hemagglutinin
HPAI	highly pathogenic avian influenza
IAV	influenza A virus
IIV	inactivated influenza vaccine
LAIV	live-attenuated influenza vaccine
LPAI	low pathogenic avian influenza
mAb	monoclonal antibody
NA	neuraminidase
NAI	neuraminidase inhibitors
PMO	phosphorodiamidate morpholino oligomer
QIV	quadrivalent influenza vaccine
RNA	ribo nucleic acid
SIV	swine influenza virus
WHO	World Health Organization

Author details

Clement Meseko[1]*, Binod Kumar[2] and Melvin Sanicas[3]

*Address all correspondence to: cameseko@yahoo.com

1 Regional Centre for Animal Influenza and Transboundary Diseases, National Veterinary Research Institute, Vom, Nigeria

2 Department of Microbiology and Immunology, Chicago Medical School, Rosalind Franklin University of Medicine and Science, North Chicago, IL, USA

3 Sanofi Pasteur, Asia and JPAC Region, Singapore, Singapore

References

[1] Kumar B, Asha K, Khanna M, Ronsard L, Meseko CA, Sanicas M. The emerging influenza virus threat: Status and new prospects for its therapy and control. Archives of Virology. 2018;**163**(4):831-844

[2] Meseko CA, Odaibo GN, Olaleye DO. Detection and isolation of 2009 pandemic influenza A/H1N1 virus in commercial piggery, Lagos Nigeria. Veterinary Microbiology. 2014;**168**(1):197-201

[3] Messenger AM, Barnes AN, Gray GC. Reverse zoonotic disease transmission (zooanthroponosis): A systematic review of seldom-documented human biological threats to animals. PLoS One. 2014;**9**(2):e89055

[4] Alexander DJ. A review of avian influenza in different bird species. Veterinary Microbiology. 2000;**74**(1-2):3-13

[5] Centre for Disease Control (CDC). Types of Influenza Viruses 2017. Available from: https://www.cdc.gov/flu/about/viruses/types.htm

[6] Tong S, Zhu X, Li Y, Shi M, Zhang J, Bourgeois M, et al. New world bats harbor diverse influenza A viruses. PLoS Pathogens. 2013;**9**(10):e1003657

[7] El Moussi A, Ledesma J, Ben Hadj Kacem MA, Pozo F, Cuevas MT, Hamdoun M, et al. Haemagglutinin D222G mutation found in a fatal case of pandemic (H1N1) flu in Tunisia. Archives of Virology. 2012;**157**(9):1813-1814

[8] Bodewes R, Bestebroer TM, van der Vries E, Verhagen JH, Herfst S, Koopmans MP, et al. Avian influenza A(H10N7) virus-associated mass deaths among harbor seals. Emerging Infectious Diseases. 2015;**21**(4):720-722

[9] Lupiani B, Reddy SM. The history of avian influenza. Comparative Immunology, Microbiology and Infectious Diseases. 2009;**32**(4):311-323

[10] Shope RE. The incidence of neutralizing antibodies for swine influenza virus in the sera of human beings of different ages. The Journal of Experimental Medicine. 1936;**63**(5): 669-684

[11] Taubenberger JK, Reid AH, Krafft AE, Bijwaard KE, Fanning TG. Initial genetic characterization of the 1918 "Spanish" influenza virus. Science. 1997;**275**(5307):1793-1796

[12] Taubenberger JK, Morens DM. 1918 influenza: The mother of all pandemics. Emerging Infectious Diseases. 2006;**12**(1):15-22

[13] Weingartl HM, Albrecht RA, Lager KM, Babiuk S, Marszal P, Neufeld J, et al. Experimental infection of pigs with the human 1918 pandemic influenza virus. Journal of Virology. 2009;**83**(9):4287-4296

[14] Nelson MI, Vincent AL. Reverse zoonosis of influenza to swine: New perspectives on the human-animal interface. Trends in Microbiology. 2015;**23**(3):142-153

[15] Taubenberger JK, Reid AH, Lourens RM, Wang R, Jin G, Fanning TG. Characterization of the 1918 influenza virus polymerase genes. Nature. 2005;**437**(7060):889-893

[16] Garten RJ, Davis CT, Russell CA, Shu B, Lindstrom S, Balish A, et al. Antigenic and genetic characteristics of swine-origin 2009 A (H1N1) influenza viruses circulating in humans. Science. 2009;**325**(5937):197-201

[17] Gao R, Cao B, Hu Y, Feng Z, Wang D, Hu W, et al. Human infection with a novel avian-origin influenza A (H7N9) virus. The New England Journal of Medicine. 2013;**368**(20): 1888-1897

[18] Reperant LA, Moesker FM, Osterhaus AD. Influenza: From zoonosis to pandemic. ERJ Open Research. 2016;**2**(1)

[19] World Health Organization. Cumulative number of confirmed human cases for avian influenza A(H5N1) reported to WHO, 2003-2017

[20] Webster RG, Bean WJ, Gorman OT, Chambers TM, Kawaoka Y. Evolution and ecology of influenza A viruses. Microbiological Reviews. 1992;**56**(1):152-179

[21] Peiris JS, de Jong MD, Guan Y. Avian influenza virus (H5N1): A threat to human health. Clinical Microbiology Reviews. 2007;**20**(2):243-267

[22] Beigel JH, Farrar J, Han AM, Hayden FG, Hyer R, de Jong MD, et al. Avian influenza A (H5N1) infection in humans. The New England Journal of Medicine. 2005;**353**(13): 1374-1385

[23] Klenk HD, Garten W. Host cell proteases controlling virus pathogenicity. Trends in Microbiology. 1994;**2**(2):39-43

[24] Walker JA, Sakaguchi T, Matsuda Y, Yoshida T, Kawaoka Y. Location and character of the cellular enzyme that cleaves the hemagglutinin of a virulent avian influenza virus. Virology. 1992;**190**(1):278-287

[25] Akanbi OB, Meseko CA, Odita CI, Shittu I, Rimfa AG, Ugbe D, et al. Epidemiology and clinicopathological manifestation of resurgent highly pathogenic avian influenza (H5N1) virus in Nigeria, 2015. Nigerian Veterinary Journal. 2015;**37**(3):175-186

[26] Richard M, Herfst S, van den Brand JM, Lexmond P, Bestebroer TM, Rimmelzwaan GF, et al. Low virulence and lack of airborne transmission of the dutch highly pathogenic avian influenza virus H5N8 in ferrets. PLoS One. 2015;**10**(6):e0129827

[27] World Health Organization. Influenza: Monthly Risk Assessment Summary; 2017

[28] Li M, Zhao N, Luo J, Li Y, Chen L, Ma J, et al. Genetic characterization of continually evolving highly pathogenic H5N6 influenza viruses in China, 2012-2016. Frontiers in Microbiology. 2017;**8**:260

[29] Avian Influenza, Human (07): CHINA (JIANGSU) H7N4, First report [press release]. 2018

[30] Meseko C, Olaleye D, Capua I, Cattoli G. Swine influenza in sub-saharan Africa–current knowledge and emerging insights. Zoonoses and Public Health. 2014;**61**(4):229-237

[31] Dawood FS, Iuliano AD, Reed C, Meltzer MI, Shay DK, Cheng PY, et al. Estimated global mortality associated with the first 12 months of 2009 pandemic influenza A H1N1 virus circulation: A modelling study. The Lancet Infectious Diseases. 2012;**12**(9):687-695

[32] Uyeki TM, Cox NJ. Global concerns regarding novel influenza A (H7N9) virus infections. The New England Journal of Medicine. 2013;**368**(20):1862-1864

[33] Bangaru S, Nieusma T, Kose N, Thornburg NJ, Finn JA, Kaplan BS, et al. Recognition of influenza H3N2 variant virus by human neutralizing antibodies. JCI Insight. 2016;**1**(10)

[34] Wong KK, Greenbaum A, Moll ME, Lando J, Moore EL, Ganatra R, et al. Outbreak of influenza A (H3N2) variant virus infection among attendees of an agricultural fair, Pennsylvania, USA, 2011. Emerging Infectious Diseases. 2012;**18**(12):1937-1944

[35] Mena I, Nelson MI, Quezada-Monroy F, Dutta J, Cortes-Fernandez R, Lara-Puente JH, et al. Origins of the 2009 H1N1 influenza pandemic in swine in Mexico. eLife. 2016:5

[36] Potter CW. A history of influenza. Journal of Applied Microbiology. 2001;**91**(4):572-579

[37] Drake JW. Rates of spontaneous mutation among RNA viruses. Proceedings of the National Academy of Sciences of the United States of America. 1993;**90**(9):4171-4175

[38] Khanna M, Kumar P, Choudhary K, Kumar B, Vijayan VK. Emerging influenza virus: A global threat. Journal of Biosciences. 2008;**33**(4):475-482

[39] Khanna M, Kumar B, Gupta N, Kumar P, Gupta A, Vijayan VK, et al. Pandemic swine influenza virus (H1N1): A threatening evolution. Indian Journal of Microbiology. 2009;**49**(4):365-369

[40] Nicholson KG, Wood JM, Zambon M. Influenza. Lancet. 2003;**362**(9397):1733-1745

[41] Wang X, Jiang H, Wu P, Uyeki TM, Feng L, Lai S, et al. Epidemiology of avian influenza A H7N9 virus in human beings across five epidemics in mainland China, 2013-17: An epidemiological study of laboratory-confirmed case series. The Lancet Infectious Diseases. 2017;**17**(8):822-832

[42] Burke DF, Smith DJ. A recommended numbering scheme for influenza A HA subtypes. PLoS One. 2014;**9**(11):e112302

[43] Xiong X, Martin SR, Haire LF, Wharton SA, Daniels RS, Bennett MS, et al. Receptor binding by an H7N9 influenza virus from humans. Nature. 2013;**499**(7459):496-499

[44] Zaraket H, Bridges OA, Duan S, Baranovich T, Yoon SW, Reed ML, et al. Increased acid stability of the hemagglutinin protein enhances H5N1 influenza virus growth in the upper respiratory tract but is insufficient for transmission in ferrets. Journal of Virology. 2013;**87**(17):9911-9922

[45] Herfst S, Schrauwen EJ, Linster M, Chutinimitkul S, de Wit E, Munster VJ, et al. Airborne transmission of influenza A/H5N1 virus between ferrets. Science. 2012;**336**(6088): 1534-1541

[46] Zhang Q, Shi J, Deng G, Guo J, Zeng X, He X, et al. H7N9 influenza viruses are transmissible in ferrets by respiratory droplet. Science. 2013;**341**(6144):410-414

[47] Sutton TC, Finch C, Shao H, Angel M, Chen H, Capua I, et al. Airborne transmission of highly pathogenic H7N1 influenza virus in ferrets. Journal of Virology. 2014;**88**(12): 6623-6635

[48] Schrauwen EJ, Richard M, Burke DF, Rimmelzwaan GF, Herfst S, Fouchier RA. Amino acid substitutions that affect receptor binding and stability of the hemagglutinin of influenza A/H7N9 virus. Journal of Virology. 2016;**90**(7):3794-3799

[49] Mehle A, Doudna JA. Adaptive strategies of the influenza virus polymerase for replication in humans. Proceedings of the National Academy of Sciences of the United States of America. 2009;**106**(50):21312-21316

[50] Yamada S, Hatta M, Staker BL, Watanabe S, Imai M, Shinya K, et al. Biological and structural characterization of a host-adapting amino acid in influenza virus. PLoS Pathogens. 2010;**6**(8):e1001034

[51] Li W, Lee HHY, Li RF, Zhu HM, Yi G, Peiris JSM, et al. The PB2 mutation with lysine at 627 enhances the pathogenicity of avian influenza (H7N9) virus which belongs to a non-zoonotic lineage. Scientific Reports. 2352;**7**(1):2017

[52] McAuley JL, Zhang K, McCullers JA. The effects of influenza A virus PB1-F2 protein on polymerase activity are strain specific and do not impact pathogenesis. Journal of Virology. 2010;**84**(1):558-564

[53] Richard M, de Graaf M, Herfst S. Avian influenza A viruses: From zoonosis to pandemic. Future Virology. 2014;**9**(5):513-524

[54] Taubenberger JK, Kash JC. Influenza virus evolution, host adaptation, and pandemic formation. Cell Host & Microbe. 2010;**7**(6):440-451

[55] Rambaut A, Pybus OG, Nelson MI, Viboud C, Taubenberger JK, Holmes EC. The genomic and epidemiological dynamics of human influenza A virus. Nature. 2008;**453**(7195): 615-619

[56] Landolt GA, Olsen CW. Up to new tricks - a review of cross-species transmission of influenza A viruses. Animal Health Research Reviews. 2007;**8**(1):1-21

[57] Reid AH, Taubenberger JK. The origin of the 1918 pandemic influenza virus: A continuing enigma. The Journal of General Virology. 2003;**84**(Pt 9):2285-2292

[58] Zhao G, Gu X, Lu X, Pan J, Duan Z, Zhao K, et al. Novel reassortant highly pathogenic H5N2 avian influenza viruses in poultry in China. PLoS One. 2012;**7**(9):e46183

[59] Lee YJ, Kang HM, Lee EK, Song BM, Jeong J, Kwon YK, et al. Novel reassortant influenza A(H5N8) viruses, South Korea, 2014. Emerging Infectious Diseases. 2014;**20**(6):1087-1089

[60] Lee DH, Sharshov K, Swayne DE, Kurskaya O, Sobolev I, Kabilov M, et al. Novel reassortant clade 2.3.4.4 avian influenza A(H5N8) virus in wild aquatic birds, Russia, 2016. Emerging Infectious Diseases. 2017;**23**(2):359-360

[61] Jhung MA, Nelson DI, Centers for Disease C, Prevention. Outbreaks of avian influenza A (H5N2), (H5N8), and (H5N1) among birds–United States, December 2014-January 2015. MMWR. Morbidity and Mortality Weekly Report. 2015;**64**(4):111

[62] Imai M, Watanabe T, Hatta M, Das SC, Ozawa M, Shinya K, et al. Experimental adaptation of an influenza H5 HA confers respiratory droplet transmission to a reassortant H5 HA/H1N1 virus in ferrets. Nature. 2012;**486**(7403):420-428

[63] Zhang Y, Zhang Q, Kong H, Jiang Y, Gao Y, Deng G, et al. H5N1 hybrid viruses bearing 2009/H1N1 virus genes transmit in Guinea pigs by respiratory droplet. Science. 2013;**340**(6139):1459-1463

[64] Sorrell EM, Wan H, Araya Y, Song H, Perez DR. Minimal molecular constraints for respiratory droplet transmission of an avian-human H9N2 influenza A virus. Proceedings of the National Academy of Sciences of the United States of America. 2009;**106**(18):7565-7570

[65] Kimble JB, Angel M, Wan H, Sutton TC, Finch C, Perez DR. Alternative reassortment events leading to transmissible H9N1 influenza viruses in the ferret model. Journal of Virology. 2014;**88**(1):66-71

[66] Shrestha SS, Swerdlow DL, Borse RH, Prabhu VS, Finelli L, Atkins CY, et al. Estimating the burden of 2009 pandemic influenza A (H1N1) in the United States (April 2009-April 2010). Clinical Infectious Diseases. 2011;**52**(Suppl 1):S75-S82

[67] Epperson S, Jhung M, Richards S, Quinlisk P, Ball L, Moll M, et al. Human infections with influenza A(H3N2) variant virus in the United States, 2011-2012. Clinical Infectious Diseases. 2013;**57**(Suppl 1):S4-S11

[68] Xue KS, Greninger AL, Perez-Osorio A, Bloom JD. Cooperating H3N2 influenza virus variants are not detectable in primary clinical samples. mSphere. 2018;**3**(1):e00552-17. DOI: 10.1128/mSphereDirect.00552-17

[69] Hannoun C. The evolving history of influenza viruses and influenza vaccines. Expert Review of Vaccines. 2013;**12**(9):1085-1094

[70] Vaccines against influenza WHO position paper - November 2012. Weekly Epidemiological Record. 2012;**87**(47):461-476

[71] Myers KP, Olsen CW, Setterquist SF, Capuano AW, Donham KJ, Thacker EL, et al. Are swine workers in the United States at increased risk of infection with zoonotic influenza virus? Clinical Infectious Diseases. 2006;**42**(1):14-20

[72] Manzoli L, Ioannidis JP, Flacco ME, De Vito C, Villari P. Effectiveness and harms of seasonal and pandemic influenza vaccines in children, adults and elderly: A critical review and re-analysis of 15 meta-analyses. Human Vaccines & Immunotherapeutics. 2012;**8**(7):851-862

[73] Centers for Disease Control and Prevention. Estimated Influenza Illnesses, Medical Visits, Hospitalizations, and Deaths Averted by Vaccination in the United States. 9 December 2016

[74] Nokleby H, Nicoll A. Risk groups and other target groups - preliminary ECDC guidance for developing influenza vaccination recommendations for the season 2010-11. Euro Surveillance. 2010;**15**(12):19525. https://doi.org/10.2807/ese.15.12.19525-en

[75] Grohskopf LA, Olsen SJ, Sokolow LZ, Bresee JS, Cox NJ, Broder KR, et al. Prevention and control of seasonal influenza with vaccines: Recommendations of the advisory committee on immunization practices (ACIP) -- United States, 2014-15 influenza season. MMWR. Morbidity and Mortality Weekly Report. 2014;**63**(32):691-697

[76] Rambe DS, DelGiudice G, Rossi S, Sanicas M. Safety and mechanism of action of licensed vaccine adjuvants. International Current Pharmaceutical Journal. 2015;**4**(8):420-431

[77] Coelingh KL, Luke CJ, Jin H, Talaat KR. Development of live attenuated influenza vaccines against pandemic influenza strains. Expert Review of Vaccines. 2014;**13**(7):855-871

[78] Lee YT, Kim KH, Ko EJ, Lee YN, Kim MC, Kwon YM, et al. New vaccines against influenza virus. Clinical and Experimental Vaccine Research. 2014;**3**(1):12-28

[79] Black S, Nicolay U, Vesikari T, Knuf M, Del Giudice G, Della Cioppa G, et al. Hemagglutination inhibition antibody titers as a correlate of protection for inactivated influenza vaccines in children. The Pediatric Infectious Disease Journal. 2011;**30**(12): 1081-1085

[80] Haq K, McElhaney JE. Immunosenescence: Influenza vaccination and the elderly. Current Opinion in Immunology. 2014;**29**:38-42

[81] Franco LM, Bucasas KL, Wells JM, Nino D, Wang X, Zapata GE, et al. Integrative genomic analysis of the human immune response to influenza vaccination. eLife. 2013;**2**:e00299

[82] Cox RJ. Correlates of protection to influenza virus, where do we go from here? Human Vaccines & Immunotherapeutics. 2013;**9**(2):405-408

[83] Yoo SJ, Kwon T, Lyoo YS. Challenges of influenza A viruses in humans and animals and current animal vaccines as an effective control measure. Clinical and Experimental Vaccine Research. 2018;**7**(1):1-15

[84] Hurt AC, Selleck P, Komadina N, Shaw R, Brown L, Barr IG. Susceptibility of highly pathogenic A(H5N1) avian influenza viruses to the neuraminidase inhibitors and adamantanes. Antiviral Research. 2007;**73**(3):228-231

[85] Reuman PD, Bernstein DI, Keefer MC, Young EC, Sherwood JR, Schiff GM. Efficacy and safety of low dosage amantadine hydrochloride as prophylaxis for influenza A. Antiviral Research. 1989;**11**(1):27-40

[86] Bright RA, Medina MJ, Xu X, Perez-Oronoz G, Wallis TR, Davis XM, et al. Incidence of adamantane resistance among influenza A (H3N2) viruses isolated worldwide from 1994 to 2005: A cause for concern. Lancet. 2005;**366**(9492):1175-1181

[87] Abed Y, Goyette N, Boivin G. Generation and characterization of recombinant influenza A (H1N1) viruses harboring amantadine resistance mutations. Antimicrobial Agents and Chemotherapy. 2005;**49**(2):556-559

[88] Hayden FG, Belshe RB, Clover RD, Hay AJ, Oakes MG, Soo W. Emergence and apparent transmission of rimantadine-resistant influenza A virus in families. The New England Journal of Medicine. 1989;**321**(25):1696-1702

[89] Hayden FG, Hay AJ. Emergence and transmission of influenza A viruses resistant to amantadine and rimantadine. Current Topics in Microbiology and Immunology. 1992;**176**: 119-130

[90] Ilyushina NA, Hoffmann E, Salomon R, Webster RG, Govorkova EA. Amantadine-oseltamivir combination therapy for H5N1 influenza virus infection in mice. Antiviral Therapy. 2007;**12**(3):363-370

[91] Dong G, Peng C, Luo J, Wang C, Han L, Wu B, et al. Adamantane-resistant influenza A viruses in the world (1902-2013): Frequency and distribution of M2 gene mutations. PLoS One. 2015;**10**(3):e0119115

[92] Pizzorno A, Bouhy X, Abed Y, Boivin G. Generation and characterization of recombinant pandemic influenza A (H1N1) viruses resistant to neuraminidase inhibitors. The Journal of Infectious Diseases. 2011;**203**(1):25-31

[93] Pizzorno A, Abed Y, Bouhy X, Beaulieu E, Mallett C, Russell R, et al. Impact of mutations at residue I223 of the neuraminidase protein on the resistance profile, replication level, and virulence of the 2009 pandemic influenza virus. Antimicrobial Agents and Chemotherapy. 2012;**56**(3):1208-1214

[94] Whitley RJ, Hayden FG, Reisinger KS, Young N, Dutkowski R, Ipe D, et al. Oral oseltamivir treatment of influenza in children. The Pediatric Infectious Disease Journal. 2001;**20**(2):127-133

[95] Hussain M, Galvin HD, Haw TY, Nutsford AN, Husain M. Drug resistance in influenza A virus: The epidemiology and management. Infection and Drug Resistance. 2017;**10**: 121-134

[96] Phanich J, Rungrotmongkol T, Kungwan N, Hannongbua S. Role of R292K mutation in influenza H7N9 neuraminidase toward oseltamivir susceptibility: MD and MM/PB(GB)SA study. Journal of Computer-Aided Molecular Design. 2016;**30**(10):917-926

[97] de Jong MD, Tran TT, Truong HK, Vo MH, Smith GJ, Nguyen VC, et al. Oseltamivir resistance during treatment of influenza A (H5N1) infection. The New England Journal of Medicine. 2005;**353**(25):2667-2672

[98] Earhart KC, Elsayed NM, Saad MD, Gubareva LV, Nayel A, Deyde VM, et al. Oseltamivir resistance mutation N294S in human influenza A(H5N1) virus in Egypt. Journal of Infection and Public Health. 2009;**2**(2):74-80

[99] Boltz DA, Douangngeun B, Phommachanh P, Sinthasak S, Mondry R, Obert C, et al. Emergence of H5N1 avian influenza viruses with reduced sensitivity to neuraminidase inhibitors and novel reassortants in Lao People's Democratic Republic. The Journal of General Virology. 2010;**91**(Pt 4):949-959

[100] Shionogi to present S-033188 Phase 3 CAPSTONE-1 Study Results For Treatment Of Influenza At IDWeek 2017 2017. Available from: http://www.shionogi.com/newsroom/article.html#122521

[101] Wong SS, Webby RJ. Traditional and new influenza vaccines. Clinical Microbiology Reviews. 2013;**26**(3):476-492

[102] Khanna M, Sharma S, Kumar B, Rajput R. Protective immunity based on the conserved hemagglutinin stalk domain and its prospects for universal influenza vaccine development. BioMed Research International. 2014;**2014**:546274

[103] Steel J, Lowen AC, Wang TT, Yondola M, Gao Q, Haye K, et al. Influenza virus vaccine based on the conserved hemagglutinin stalk domain. MBio. 2010;**1**(1):e00018-10. DOI: 10.1128/mBio.00018-10

[104] Schwartzman LM, Cathcart AL, Pujanauski LM, Qi L, Kash JC, Taubenberger JK. An intranasal virus-like particle vaccine broadly protects mice from multiple subtypes of influenza A virus. MBio. 2015;**6**(4):e01044

Section 4

Preparation of Vaccines Against Potential Pandemic Influenza

Chapter 4

Preparing Live Influenza Vaccines against Potential Pandemic Influenza Using Nonpathogenic Avian Influenza Viruses and Cold-Adapted Master Donor Strain

Yulia Desheva

Additional information is available at the end of the chapter

http://dx.doi.org/10.5772/intechopen.76980

Abstract

As part of an influenza pandemic preparedness program, the WHO analyzes a range of potentially pandemic influenza viruses for appropriate vaccines development. Several vaccine candidates were prepared using classical genetic reassortment, with the cold-adapted A/Leningrad/134/17/57(H2N2) (Len/17) master donor strain (MDS) which is licensed in the Russia for the live influenza vaccine (LAIV) strains type A production for adults and children. The nonpathogenic avian viruses of different subtypes were used for reassortant vaccine strains preparation. All vaccine candidates demonstrated a high reproductive capacity and cold-adapted (*ca*-) phenotype in chick embryos. In mice, the LAIV of H5N2, H7N3, and H9N2 subtypes provided protection against infection with distant influenza viruses. The immunogenicity and protective efficacy of H7N3 LAIV was also demonstrated in ferrets. The H5N2 and H7N3 vaccine candidates demonstrated the inability to reproduce in chickens, which confirms the safety of their use in areas with highly developed agriculture. When tested in clinical trials, vaccine strains of H5N2 and H7N3 subtypes induce the conversions of antibodies homologous and antigenically distant variants. The use of LAIV can be effective against highly pathogenic influenza viruses even in the case of incomplete antigenic correspondence between the vaccine strain and the infectious virus.

Keywords: live influenza vaccine, avian influenza, attenuation, reassortment, cross-protection

1. Introduction

Influenza viruses belong to the family *Orthomyxoviridae*. These are RNA-containing viruses possessing a negative fragmented genome. To date, there are four types (serotype) of influenza viruses—influenza A, B, C, and D. Influenza A viruses affect humans and a wide range of mammals (horses, pigs, dogs, wild and domestic cats, seals, ferrets) and birds (chickens, wild waterfowl, gulls, etc.). Only influenza A viruses are known as causative agents of severe epidemics and pandemics. The antigenic properties of influenza A viruses are based on two surface glycoproteins, hemagglutinin (HA) and neuraminidase (NA).

Wild waterfowl are considered as a natural reservoir of influenza A viruses which is characterized by high divergence. The 16 HA subtypes and nine NA subtypes were detected in migratory waterfowl and poultry [1]. Sometimes, avian influenza viruses overcome the interspecies barrier and infect poultry and mammals. Avian influenza viruses of subtypes H5N1, H7N3, H7N7, H7N9, and H9N2 may become pathogenic for humans and occasionally cause very severe infections. As part of an influenza pandemic preparedness program, the World Health Organization (WHO) analyzes a range of zoonotic and potentially pandemic influenza viruses for the development of appropriate vaccines as seasonal influenza vaccination does not protect against pandemic avian influenza viruses [2].

After isolation of the first influenza viruses in 1933–1936, the development of influenza vaccines in England, the United States, Australia, and in the USSR began. The development of active immunization against influenza using live attenuated vaccines was conducted in Russia under the leadership of A.A. Smorodintsev since 1937, and in the USA since 1960, where the group of H.F. Maassab also obtained cold-adapted attenuated variants of influenza viruses A and B. At present, two types of LAIVs are commercially available. The first, based on cold-adapted master donor viruses (MDVs) A/Leningrad/134/17/57 (H2N2) and B/USSR/60/69 [3–5], was licensed in 1987 for the people 3 years and older as Ultravac (Microgen, Russia). The second, known as FluMist based on cold-adapted MDVs, A/Ann Arbor/6/60ca (H2N2), and B/Ann Arbor/1/66ca, was licensed in 2003 (MedImmune, Inc., USA). FluMist is used for the prevention of influenza in persons younger than 49 and older than 2 years of age [6]. According to World Health Organization (WHO), vaccination prevents influenza in 80–90% of vaccinated people, and the economic effect of influenza vaccinations is 10–20 times higher than the cost of vaccination. In the past 10 years, attention was paid due to the advantages of LAIV that cause the formation of systemic and strong local (secretory) immunity. By contrast, parenteral inactivated influenza vaccines (IIV) stimulate mainly the formation of serum strain-specific antibodies which offer only limited protection against newly emerging viruses [7]. Intranasal implementation of LAIV produces immune response similar to natural infection and therefore induces an earlier, broader, and more long-lasting protection than inactivated vaccines [8]. Besides, the cost of live vaccine is five times less than inactivated vaccine, and the productivity of the biotechnological production process is significantly higher which is also important in the event of pandemic.

2. Avian influenza in humans

Most avian viruses are initially low virulent for birds, causing only transient asymptomatic intestinal infections in wild waterfowl [9]. Viruses of subtypes H5 and H7 can be widespread among poultry, while acquiring the increased pathogenicity. This was observed during outbreaks caused by H5N2 viruses in 1983 or 1994–1995 in North America [10, 11], subtype H7 (H7N7 or H7N2)—in Europe and in Australia [12]. For the first time, "bird plague," a disease caused (as is now known) by highly pathogenic influenza viruses, was described in 1878 during an outbreak among chickens in Italy. The outbreak causative agent was isolated in 1902 (virus A/Chicken/Brescia/1902 (H7N7)). During similar outbreaks, repeatedly observed in Europe and around the world, several other viruses of H7 subtype were isolated. In 1955, those viruses were identified as belonging to a group of influenza viruses [13]. The first of the highly pathogenic (HP) viruses of the H5N3 subtype—the A/Tern/South Africa/61—was isolated in 1961 [14]. HP avian influenza viruses can cause a mass death of chickens in a short time as a result of dissemination of infection in poultry with rapidly progressive neurologic symptoms, diarrhea, and fatal outcome. Until 1997, there was no obvious evidence of direct infection of humans with avian viruses. Nevertheless, serological studies revealed the presence of antibodies against avian viruses of various subtypes in human sera in southern China, Hong Kong, and East Asia, indicating exposure of some people to avian influenza viruses [15].

2.1. H5N1 influenza viruses

For the first time, attention to H5 avian influenza viruses as possible pandemic agents was brought in May 1997 in Hong Kong during a mass outbreak among chickens when the avian virus H5N1 was isolated from a child who died from viral pneumonia [16]. To the end of 1997, an infection with the virus H5N1 similar to poultry viruses identified in the region was confirmed in another 17 people, five of whom died [17].

It is possible that before the appearance of the virus H5N1 in humans, a series of reassortments during the circulation of a number of precursor viruses in birds have occurred. Thus, HA of H5N1 viruses isolated from humans were almost identical to those of the A/Goose/Guandong/1/96 (H5N1) [18], and NA may have been acquired from the virus H6N1 [24]. It is assumed that the internal genes were borrowed from the same H6N1 virus or H9N2 A/Qail/Hong Kong/G1/97 (H9N2) influenza viruses during transmission from waterfowl to quails and chickens [19].

The mechanisms of avian influenza viruses "step-by-step" adaptation to new hosts are well characterized [20]. The change in host cell specificity and the increase in the pathogenicity of influenza viruses can be influenced either by amino acid substitutions in the receptor binding site of HA or by substitutions affecting the conformation and steric availability of this center. In particular, this can be influenced by changes in the number of glycosylation sites or their localization. High pathogenicity of avian influenza viruses in mammals is polygenic in nature. The HA of H5 or H7 HP viruses with a polybasic cleavage site is known as a primary virulence factor, although the unusual severity of clinical manifestations during human infection with influenza H5N1 viruses can also be associated with mutations in internal proteins (PB1-F2, PB2) and non-structural (NS) proteins.

From 1997 to 2001, the HA of H5N1 viruses remained antigenically conserved, although, since 2003, there has been an unusually high level of H5N1 viruses evolution. The HP H5N1 viruses isolated from poultry and humans separated into three branches that differ antigenically and genetically [21]. During the outbreak in 2005 on Lake Qinghai, a number of HP H5N1 viruses were isolated from wild waterfowl [22]. This may indicate a reverse drift of similar viruses from poultry to wild birds, which was not observed previously. Along with H5 HA evolution, the extensive reassortment of avian influenza viruses in birds in China resulted in new H5 viruses possessing different NA subtypes (H5N2, H5N5, H5N6, and H5N8) and internal protein genes. In 2014, HA gene segments of H5N1, H5N2, H5N5, H5N6, and H5N8 were designated as clade 2.3.4.4., which were detected in birds in 40 countries in Africa, Asia, and Europe [23].

WHO has consistently recorded cases of human infection caused by HP influenza H5N1 virus, many of which had fatal outcomes. The clinical features of human infection caused highly pathogenic H5N1 viruses are characterized not only by primary viral pneumonia but also by complications with acute distress syndrome and poly-organ lesions [24].

At present, cases of human infection with the avian influenza H5N1 virus were decreased compared to the early 2000s. From 2003 to 2009, 468 cases of this disease were registered in 16 countries, mainly in Vietnam, China, Indonesia, Thailand, and Egypt. In 2010–2014, the number of cases was two times decreased (233 people). In 2016, the virus continued to infect people in only one country—Egypt (10 cases, three of them with a fatal outcome). In 2017, again in Egypt three cases were recorded, one of which was fatal. Thus, even when the absolute number of cases was decreased, mortality remains extremely high. In total, according to WHO data, by mid-2017, 859 people were infected with influenza H5N1, 453 (53%) from which died [25].

During the outbreak in Hong Kong in 1997, there was no direct evidence of a sustained human-to-human transmission of H5N1 viruses, although antibodies against H5 viruses were detected in 3.7% of physicians who had contact with H5-infected patients [26]. In 2008, transmission of an infection with avian influenza H5N1 from a son to his father was registered in China [27]. Under conditions of the continuous appearance HP H5N1 viruses in the humans, there is a risk of such a transmission during close contacts.

2.2. H7N9 influenza viruses

On March 31, 2013, the first three cases of human infection with the avian influenza H7N9 virus were registered in China. In all three cases, an infection of the respiratory tract was complicated with severe pneumonia. Two patients died, the third was in a critical condition for a long time, but recovered. Since then, the number of laboratory-confirmed cases in China has increased every day. In addition to severe and lethal cases, the sero-diagnostics methods have proved the asymptomatic course of the disease in workers of poultry farms. From March

2013, there were 1566 cases of avian influenza H7N9 in the world, of which 613 (39%) were fatal [28]. At the same time, 88% of the infected developed severe pneumonia, 68% was hospitalized in the intensive care unit. Mortality in different years ranged from 31 to 39%.

Experts believe that the virus H7N9 is not likely transmitted from person to person, but can spread with prolonged contact, especially when people care for sick family members. Moreover, the reassortment of several viruses is also not excluded. Genome analysis of human-isolated H7N9 viruses has shown adaptive evolution and convergent changes in eight viral genes, including sites in the PB2 gene (Q591K, E627K, and D701N), in HA (R156K, V202A, and L244Q), and in NA (R289K). These substitutions are known as playing a role in crossing species barriers from avian to human [29].

2.3. H9N2 influenza viruses

The H9N2 influenza viruses readily transmit from birds to animals and humans due to the easy appearance of variants that have an affinity for sialic receptors in mammals [30]. Sero-epidemiological studies revealed antibodies to viruses H9N2 among 15% of poultry workers in China [31]. Viruses H9N2 were isolated from people with symptoms of respiratory infection in Hong Kong and China from 1997 to 2009 [32] belonging mainly to the antigenic G1 line, unlike other H9N2 viruses isolated from swine and poultry belonging to the antigenic variety G9 [33]. Phylogenetic analysis showed that after 1994, Eurasian H9N2 after complex genetic reassortment of G1 and G9 viruses circulating among wild and domestic birds formed several antigenic lines [34]. The H9N2 viruses, which caused human cases, were not HP as they did not possess highly cleavable HA and were not highly virulent for poultry, although molecular analysis demonstrated similarity of genes for internal proteins with HP H5N1 viruses, which caused an outbreak among people in 1997 [35]. Due to the fact that the avian influenza viruses of the H9 subtype are transmitted to humans, have genetic similarity to the H5N1 viruses, and are widespread in Asia, Europe, and the Middle East, the WHO has included H9N2 vaccine development in the overall plan for pre-pandemic training [36].

2.4. H6N1 influenza viruses

Serological studies in Southern China revealed that 13% of people from different provinces have antibodies to the influenza virus of H6 subtype [37]. Phylogenic analysis of influenza A viruses indicates that the closely related genes coding the internal proteins could be found in influenza A viruses of different subtypes and that the reassortment between the avian and human influenza viruses is possible [38]. It was also shown that some of the fragments of the NP and NA genes of highly pathogenic H5N1 viruses originated from the H6 virus of wild ducks [18, 39]. Therefore, the avian influenza viruses of H6N1 subtype may represent a potential danger for humans.

Thus, various avian influenza viruses can pose a threat to humans that necessitates the development of a corresponding vaccine strain for the protection of humans from possible infection. As part of an influenza pandemic preparedness program, the WHO monitors the number of zoonotic and potentially pandemic influenza viruses to schedule candidates for the development of appropriate vaccines [40].

3. Development of live influenza vaccines against potentially pandemic avian influenza

The LAIVs preparation against potentially pandemic avian influenza viruses is conducted in two directions: the preparation of vaccine strains using classical genetic reassortment in chick embryos or through reverse genetics (RG) technique. The first attenuated A/Ann Arbor/6/60 (H2N2)-based vaccine strains were obtained by reverse genetics shortly after H5 influenza outbreaks in Hong Kong in 1997 [41].

The vaccine candidates containing internal genes from the attenuation donor, and the surface antigens from viruses A/Hong Kong/156/97 (H5N1) or A/Hong Kong/483/97 (H5N1) with RG-modified HA demonstrated an attenuated phenotype for ferrets and chickens. Both reassortants caused seroconversions in chickens, which confirm the sensitivity of chickens to these vaccine strains despite the *att*-phenotype [42]. By RG methods, three reassortant strains based on the A/Ann Arbor/6/60 (H2N2) were prepared in the Vero cell line [43]. As a source of surface antigens, viruses H5N1 of 1997, 2003, and 2004 years of isolation with RG-modified HA were used. It was shown that a double immunization with LAIV from a strain isolated in 1997 completely protected mice from infection with later "wild" isolates, including the isolate obtained in 2005—A/Indonesia/05/2005 (H5N1). The use of HP viruses requires increased biosecurity level laboratories, certified cell lines, and RG techniques. The HP avian viruses found in nature cannot be used directly to prepare influenza vaccines because they would not grow in eggs and might be dangerous to people. The RG-modified viruses do not cause severe illness in birds and that also will grow well in chicken eggs (so that vaccine manufacturers can use it to produce vaccine). An alternative approach is to use low pathogenic surrogate viruses that show antigenic similarity to HP viruses. In this regard, the identification of non-pathogenic variants, which are antigenically close to potentially pandemic strains, may be very important.

Another vaccine candidate based on A/Ann Arbor/6/60, containing HA and NA from virus A/duck/Hokkaido/69/2000 (H5N3), A/chicken/Hong Kong/G9/97 (H9N2), or A/Chicken/British Columbia/CN-6/04 (H7N3) was prepared by classical genetic reassortment methods in the chick embryos (CE) [44–46]. The vaccine strains exhibited *ts*-, *ca*-, and *att*-phenotype and provided protection against infection with the wild-type virus in mice and ferrets.

3.1. Development of reassortant vaccine strains based on a/Leningrad/134/17/57 (H2N2) MDV

To prepare vaccines based on A/Leningrad/134/17/57 (H2N2) MDV, several non-pathogenic avian viruses of different subtypes (A/duck/Potsdam/1402–6/1986 (H5N2), A/mallard /The Netherlands/12/2000 (H7N3), A/Hong Kong/1073/99 (H9N2), A/quail/Hong Kong/G1/1997 (H9N2), and A/herring gull/Sarma/51 s/2006 (H6N1)) were used. The HP avian influenza viruses of subtypes H5 and H7 contain a HA insertion from several positively charged amino acid residues (lysine and arginine) in the proteolytic cleavage site [47], which causes effective cleavage of HA by intracellular proteases expressed in most organs and tissues of birds and mammals. Unlike HP avian influenza viruses, non-pathogenic viruses contain a single arginine residue (R) in the cleavage site [44]. For non-pathogenic viruses proteolytic activation, the presence of trypsin-like enzymes is required, which is expressed by a limited range of cells and is found in the airways.

The reassortant vaccine strains were prepared in the Virology Department, Institute of Experimental Medicine, using classical genetic reassortment in CE as previously described [48]. The H5N2 reassortant virus inherited only the HA gene from the H5N2 parent virus, and the remaining seven genes from the Len/17 MDV (7,1 genome composition) [49]. The reassortants of subtypes H7N3, H9N2, and H6N1 inherited the HA and NA from parental avian influenza viruses (6,2 genome composition). All the reassortant strains were studied for temperature-sensitive (*ts*-) and cold-adapted (*ca*-) phenotype [49–52]. For those purposes, the reassortant viruses were propagated in CE for 2 days at 25, 34, and 40°C. The yield of "wild-type" avian influenza viruses at 40°C was the same or greater than at 34°C. Only when the temperature was increased to 41°C, the reproduction of these strains was partially limited. Thus, the high degree of temperature resistance of all the above viruses was demonstrated. In contrast to parental avian viruses, all vaccine candidates poorly reproduced at 40°C in titers not exceeded 1.5–1.8 $\log_{10}$ EID_{50}/ml. At the same time, these reassortant strains grew well at low temperatures. Thus, all obtained reassortants acquired the genes of internal and nonstructural proteins from the A/Leningrad/134/17/57 (H2N2) MDV inherited the *ts*- and *ca*-phenotype. The pronounced difference in optimal reproductive conditions between the temperature-resistant viruses of avian influenza and the cold-adapted attenuation donor is due to the properties of viral polymerases [53]. This difference in the temperature optimum of the parental viruses may facilitate the isolation of the reassortant viruses possessing the desired gene composition after selective passages at a lower temperature.

3.2. Immunogenicity and cross-protection in mice

The ability of LAIV to induce antibodies not only to the homologous variant subtype but also to cross-reacting antibodies to antigenically different variants including HP variants was shown in several mouse studies [50–52, 54–56].

Among all vaccine candidates based on non-pathogenic avian influenza viruses, the H6N1 LAIV was characterized by the highest HI titers in mice after a single administration (GMT = 17.4). The LAIV of H7N3 subtype raised serum antibodies not only against the homologous virus but also against H7N9, which possessed the difference of 3% in the HA amino acid sequence. In the sera from mice double-vaccinated with H7N3 LAIV, serum HI titers against H7N9 were 20–40 times higher than against H7N3 ($P < 0.05$) [56]. At the same time, local IgA levels were higher against homologous H7N3 compared with H7N9 after vaccination with LAIV. The H5N2 LAIV induced detectable HI and neutralizing antibody titers only against the homologous H5N2 virus, perhaps due to the genetic differences between H5N2 vaccine strain and infectious viruses H5N1 isolated in 1997, 2003, and 2005 (10–12% differences of the HA1 amino acid sequence).

Nevertheless, immunization using virus H5N2 of 1986 resulted in a significant level of protection in experimental infection of mice (**Figure 1**).

Data on the protective efficacy of reassortant vaccine strains against intranasal challenge with avian influenza viruses are summarized in **Table 1**. When the mice were challenged with HP H5N1 viruses following immunization with H5N2 LAIV, the infectious viruses were not isolated from nasal passages or from the brain [54, 55]. Limited reproduction of HP viruses in the respiratory tract of mice and preventing a systemic infection, including neuro-infections, are important advantages of LAIV, especially in respect with data on the neurogenic pathway of generalization of infection caused by HP H5N1 viruses [58]. The absence of nasal infection correlated with high titers of secretory virus-specific IgA viruses in nasal swabs. The local immune response of the mucous membranes of the body serves as the first and most significant barrier for many viral infections, including influenza [59]. Due to their polymeric structure, IgAs have several times higher anti-hemagglutinating and neutralizing activity compared to IgG [60] and are also more stable and more cross-reactive. In addition, IgA can interact with the surface proteins of the influenza virus intracellularly, during trans-cytosis [61]. With respect to LAIV, it is still unclear how antibody-mediated immune response is related to protective efficacy. Mechanisms of cross-immunity in influenza are mediated by several factors, among which the cellular immune response is very important. Cellular immunity is involved in virus clearance and in activating the humoral immune response. In this regard, the production of Th1 and Th2 marker cytokines *in vitro* by splenocytes from mice immunized with H5N2 LAIV and whole-virion H5N2 IIV was compared [55].

Both LAIV and IIV caused the cytokines production by splenocytes of immunized mice in response to stimulation with both whole H5N1 virus and recombinant H5 HA. While immunization with LAIV caused higher levels of IFN-γ production by splenocytes of mice stimulated with H5N1 viruses, immunization with IIV induced IL-4 and IL-10 production. Interestingly,

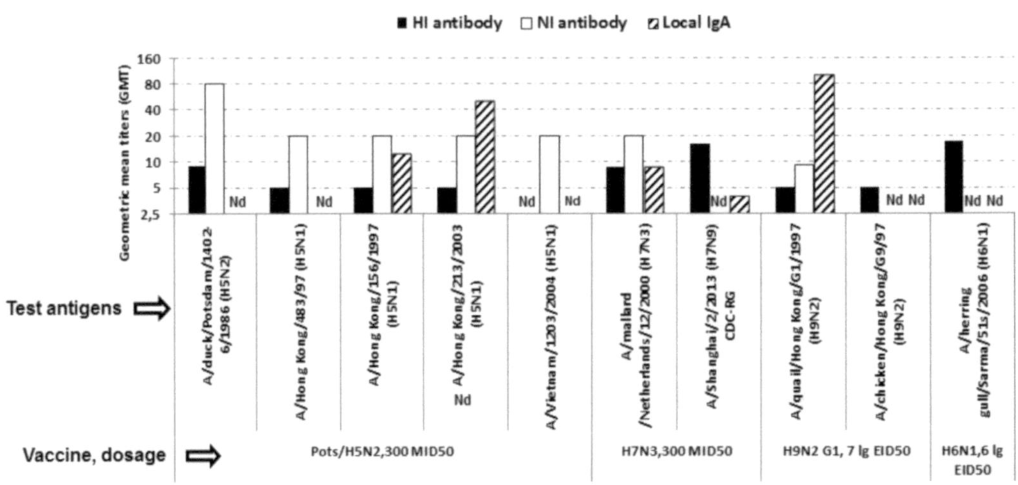

Figure 1. Influenza virus-specific serum antibodies and local IgA in mice after intranasal (i.n.) immunization with LAIV [50–52, 54–56]. *Nd, not done.

Challenge virus	Dosage	Vaccine groups	Protection				Refs.
			Virus titers ($log_{10}EID_{50}$/ml)			Lethality	
			Lung	Noses	Brain		
A/Hong Kong/483/97 (H5N1)	50 LD_{50}	H5N2 LAIV	1.9	≤0.8	≤0.8	0%	[54]
		PBS	5.9	4.0	4.3	100%	
A/Hong Kong/213/2003 (H5N1)	100 MID_{50}	H5N2 LAIV	1.8	Nd*	Nd	Na**	[54]
		PBS	5.3	Nd	Nd	Na	
A/Vietnam/1203/2004 (H5N1)	200 LD_{50}	H5N2 LAIV	1.6	0.8	0.8	0%	[55]
		PBS	6.1	4.7	4.5	100%	
A/chicken/Kurgan/02/2005 (H5N1)	27 LD_{50}	H5N2 LAIV	Nd	Nd	Nd	13%	[57]
		PBS	Nd	Nd	Nd	100%	
A/mallard/The Netherlands/12/2000 (H7N3)	7 lg EID_{50}	H7N3 LAIV	≤1.5	≤1.5	≤1.5	Na	[50]
		PBS	5.7	4.2	≤1.5	Na	[50]
A/chicken/Hong Kong/G9/97 (H9N2)	7 lg EID_{50}	H9N2 LAIV	3.4	1.1	Nd	Nd	[51]
		PBS	6.9	2.0	Nd	Nd	[51]

*Nd, not done.

**Na, not applicable.

The virus was not lethal for mice.

Table 1. Protection against infection with avian influenza viruses.

after immunization with the H2N2 MDV, the IFN-γ production by splenocyte of mice occurred only in response to stimulation with whole virus H5N1, but not purified HA. This may indicate the directivity of hetero-subtypic immunity to conserved epitopes of viral proteins [55].

3.3. Pathogenicity for chickens

Several experiments with vaccine candidates H5N2 and H7N3 were performed at Southeast Poultry Research Laboratory, GA, USA. Those studies demonstrated that the *ca*- reassortants of avian viruses adapted to a lower temperature of reproduction were unable to either infect a bird or be released into the environment. This was confirmed by the absence of virus isolation from the gastrointestinal tract of birds, as well as the impossibility in the determination of specific antibodies (**Table 2**).

A high degree of attenuation of H5N2 and H7N3 reassortants in chickens (up to a total inability) to reproduce confirms the safety for poultry farms during the production and use of such strains.

3.4. Study in primates

If the genetically homogeneous population using linear mice is the most appropriate model for assessing the molecular mechanisms of pathogenicity, the use of genetically heterogeneous

Virus	I.v. pathogenicity test*		I.n. pathogenicity and infectivity data**					Refs.
			Virus isolation on day 3 p.i.		Seroconversions (AGID).	Morbidity	Mortality	
	Morbidity	Mortality	Oropharyngeal swabs	Cloacal swabs				
Len/17	0/8	0/8	0/5	0/5	0/5	0/5	0/5	[53]
Len17/H5N2	0/8	0/8	0/5	0/5	0/5	0/5	0/5	
H5N2-wt	0/8	0/8	0/5	0/5	3/5	0/5	0/5	
Len17/H7N3	0/8	0/8	0/5	0/5	0/5	0/5	0/5	[49]
H7N3-wt	5/8	5/8	2/5($10^{1.1}$)***	1/5($10^{0.91}$)***	5/5	0/5	0/5	

*Groups of eight 5-week-old specific pathogen-free (SPF) chickens were infected intravenously (i.v.) with and observed daily for 10 days for clinical signs and death.

**Groups of five chickens were infected intranasally (i.n.) with 6 log_{10} EID_{50}/0.1 ml. The oropharyngeal and cloacal swabs were collected 3 days post infection (p.i.) and titrated in eggs for assessing viral replication. The chickens were observed for clinical signs of disease and death for 14 days. To determine infectivity, sera were collected 21 days p.i. and tested for the presence of antibodies by agar gel immunodiffusion (AGID) test.

***Mean virus titers (EID_{50}/0.1 ml).

Table 2. Pathogenicity and infectivity data for chickens.

animals (ferrets, primates) better allows one to assess the effect of natural host defense factors in mammalian infection by avian influenza viruses. The use of primates is one of the most promising areas in the study of human infectious pathology. The evolutionary relationship and biological similarity between humans and monkeys make them unique objects in the modeling of infectious diseases. However, the lower primates, while remaining closest to humans than other mammals, differ significantly in physiological characteristics from them. In experiments on the hybridization of nuclear DNA, it has been established that the similarity of man to chimpanzee reaches 90–98%, with lower monkeys—50–75% whereas in rodents, this index is not more than 20% (unpublished data).

The use of lower primates as models makes it possible to establish the duration and sequence of biochemical, metabolic, and physiological responses in the course of the development of the disease, which are then used to evaluate various preventive and therapeutic measures [62]. The use of primates for the modeling of the pathogenesis of influenza H5N1 in people of preclinical evaluation of vaccine preparations by a group of scientists from The Netherlands is described [63].

Before the clinical trials, the safety, immunogenicity, and protective properties of the LAIV based on strain A/17/duck/Potsdam/86/92 (H5N2) were studied by intranasal immunization of Java macaques [64]. None of the four monkeys immunized with H5N2 LAIV at a dose of 6.9 log_{10} EID_{50}/ml showed no adverse reactions with either temperature or behavioral changes or weight loss. The vaccine virus multiplied in the upper respiratory tract and was isolated in two of four monkeys, on days 3–5 after the first vaccination with the maximum titer of 4.2 lg EID50/ml. The absence of viremia and a temperature reaction in the same period indicates the local immunization process. In three of four monkeys, double immunization caused neutralizing antibodies to H5 viruses in titers 1:40–1:160. Twenty-one days after the end of the immunization cycle, the animals were infected in a combined method using intratracheal and intranasal administration of 7.5 lg EID_{50}/ml primate-adapted influenza virus A/Chicken/Kurgan/2/05 (H5N1). According to the summary data on clinical reactions and virus isolation from the respiratory tract, the vaccine protected at least 50% of immunized animals against the H5N1 infection.

3.5. Study of the H5N2 and H7N3 reassortants in phase I clinical trials

The randomized, double-blinded, placebo-controlled phase I trials were conducted in healthy adults at the St. Petersburg Institute of Influenza [65, 66]. Both H5N2 and H7N3 LAIV were safe for volunteers. In the genome of the isolated vaccine virus, all the mutations known for the MDV were conserved [65, 66]. Data on the LAIV when used in humans confirm the concept of attenuation of influenza viruses by reassortment with MDV and association of the ca- phenotype with an attenuation for people. For the vaccine virus isolation from the nasal washes, two to three passages were required on MDCK cell culture, indicating a very low content of the virus. These data confirmed LAIV implementation safety for contact persons.

The post-vaccination antibody response was assessed using the HI test, which is still posing as the "gold standard" for the evaluation of influenza vaccine immunogenicity, the micro-neutralization (MN) test which is supposed to be more sensitive compared to the HI in the detection of serum antibodies after immunization against potential pandemic subtypes. Local IgA response in nasal washes was estimated using ELISA (**Figure 2**).

According to the results of three tests, more than 80% of the vaccinated subjects responded to immunization with a significant increase in serum or local antibodies [65, 66]. Moreover, after double vaccination with H5N2 LAIV, 30.8% of vaccinated volunteers responded to the HA antigen of the A/Indonesia/05/2005xPR8 IBCDC-RG (H5N1). When serum samples of volunteers vaccinated with H7N3 LAIV were tested for the anti-H7N9 HI antibodies, the

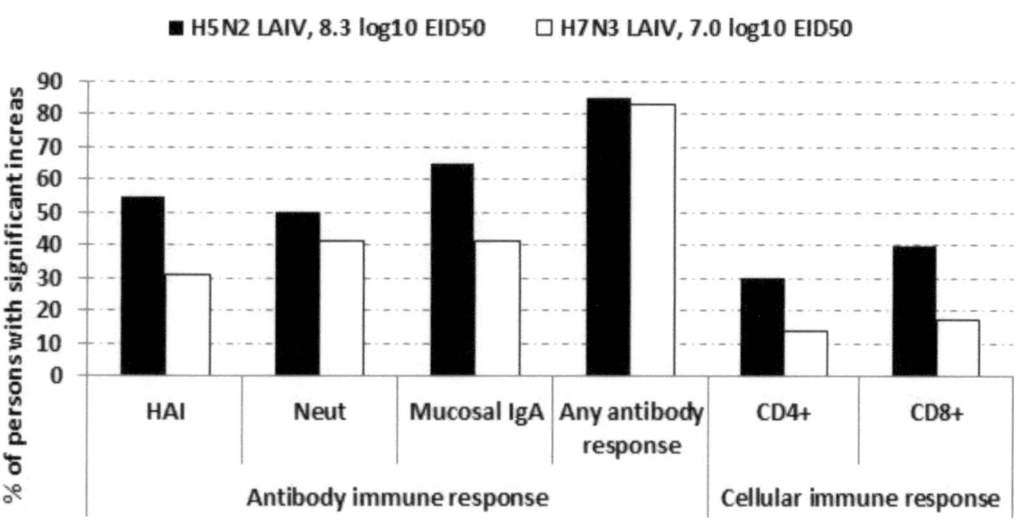

Figure 2. Immunogenicity of H5N2 and H7N3 LAIV in volunteers after boost immunization [65–67].

Vaccine	Groups	NI data				Ref.
		Number of ≥2-fold antibody rises	Geometric mean titers (GMT)		GMT fold-rise	
			Before vaccination	After revaccination		
LAIV H5N2 (6.9 log_{10} EID_{50}/0.5 ml)	LAIV	6 (33.3)	5.0	9.9	2.0*	[71]
	Placebo	0 (0)	9.9	7.5	0	

*P < 0.05.

Table 3. Serum NA-inhibiting antibodies against H5N2 LAIV 21 days after second vaccination.

seroconversions were found among 44.8% of vaccinated persons [67]. These data indicate the substantial level of cross-reactive antibodies induced by LAIV against distant avian influenza viruses. The two doses of LAIV raised both CD4 and CD8 T-memory-cell responses in peripheral blood of healthy volunteers on day 21 after boost immunization [67].

Previously, when studying the immunogenicity of inactivated vaccines based on potentially pandemic avian influenza viruses, both the experiment and the clinical trials showed a low immunogenicity of such preparations, according to generally accepted criteria for seroconversion of HI antibodies. The European Committee for the Control of Medicines has established the following criteria for the immunogenicity of vaccine preparations based on both epidemic and potentially pandemic influenza viruses: the multiplicity of antibody growths of at least 2.5 for individuals 18–60 years old and the development of reliable seroconversion in 40% of the vaccinated [68]. Obviously, the detection of only strain-specific HI antibodies is not sufficient to fully characterize the immunogenicity of the LAIV [69]. Moreover, it remains unclear what antibody titer can be considered protective against potentially pandemic viruses—1:20 or 1:40. Recently, it was shown that neuraminidase-inhibiting (NI) antibody titers better correlate with protection and can be an independent predictor of reduction of influenza disease severity [70]. Therefore, neuraminidase immunity should be considered when studying susceptibility after vaccination as a critical target in future influenza vaccine platforms. In this connection, the NI antibodies in the sera of volunteers after H5N2 immunization were estimated (**Table 3**). The two doses of the monovalent LAIV H5N2 raised a statistically significant increase in the NI antibodies against vaccine strain. More than twofold increase in antibodies was obtained among 19.5–33.3% of those vaccinated. The MN test and NI assay titers in the same sera of the vaccinated volunteers were 73.2% corresponded and suggested a statistically significant correlation between the values in antibody titers revealed in both tests (p = 0.04).

4. Conclusions

- The use of non-pathogenic avian viruses as a source of surface antigens combined with the use of cold-adapted "donors" of attenuation can be a significant advantage in the development of vaccine strains for LAIV against potentially pandemic influenza using classical genetic reassortment in CE. Low pathogenic avian influenza viruses do not contain a polybasic amino acid insertion in the cleavage site and therefore do not require modification by reverse genetics methods prior to reassortment.

- A high degree of attenuation of the reassortants of subtypes H5N2 and H7N3 in chickens, up to a total inability to reproduce, confirms the safety for poultry farms during the production and use of such strains. The high yield of the obtained reassortants in the CE makes it possible to produce a large amount of viral material, which allows their use for the production of both LAIV and IIV.
- In preclinical and clinical studies, LAIV based on non-pathogenic avian influenza viruses causes the formation of systemic and secretory antibodies including those against antigenically distant viruses. In animal models, LAIV based on non-pathogenic avian influenza viruses provided protection against HP variants that appeared much later. Protection from lethal infection with HP viruses was observed even in the absence of HI antibodies. This suggests that the use of LAIV may be effective against HP influenza viruses even in the case of incomplete antigenic correspondence between the vaccine strain and the infectious virus.
- In general, studies in mice represent an adequate preclinical model for studying the properties of reassortants of non-pathogenic avian influenza viruses, since data on the safety, immunogenicity, and cross-reactivity of post-vaccinal antibodies obtained in mice were confirmed in clinical trials.
- In the clinical trials of LAIV of potentially pandemic subtypes, the detection of only strain-specific HI antibodies is not sufficient to fully characterize the positive effect of immunization on the stimulation of antiviral immunity, which in this case is mediated by a variety of other factors, both humoral and cellular.

5. Future perspectives

In the face of a pandemic threat, only live vaccines can eliminate the risk of losses from increased morbidity and mortality, as it was demonstrated in the cases with smallpox eradication and polio control. The conducted studies clearly showed that the classical genetic reassortment method allows obtaining high-yield, harmless and immunogenic LAIVs on the basis of an attenuated donor virus. In the post-pandemic period, when the direct threat of infection recedes, the main task is the search for optimal regimens for the use of new pandemic vaccines, including (1) the possibility of including such vaccine strains in the composition of polyvalent live vaccines; (2) prime-boost schemes using both LAIV and IIV; (3) the development of recommendations for vaccination of people with an increased risk of influenza infection complications; (4) a comprehensive study of the immune mechanisms of vaccination with influenza vaccines against emerging variant viruses; (5) the development of the most reliable and standardized assays to measure post-vaccination immune response.

Currently, the FluMist LAIV, which was withdrawn from use in the USA and Europe in 2015 due to reduced LAIV effectiveness against A/H1N1pdm09, was returned to the practice by the CDC's Advisory Committee on Immunization Practices (ACIP) (http://www.cidrap.umn.edu/news-perspective/2018/02/cdc-vaccine-panel-brings-back-flumist-2018-19-season). It was noted that after the replacement of A/H1N1pdm09 vaccine strain in the quadrivalent LAIV, an immune response was achieved similar to that of highly immunogenic seasonal A/H1N1 viruses circulating before 2009. Therefore, at present, much attention is paid to influenza vaccine strategies that target more broadly reactive antibodies which also apply to potentially pandemic vaccine strains.

Acknowledgements

The author is grateful to the postgraduate student of the Institute of Experimental Medicine Ivan Sychev for the editorial changes. The author also expresses thanks to the Microgen and PATH with the support of which the described studies were performed.

Conflict of interest

The author confirms that this manuscript content has no conflict of interest.

Abbreviations

AGID	agar gel immunodiffusion
CE	chick embryos
ca-	cold-adapted
EID_{50}	fifty percent egg infectious dose
HI	hemagglutination inhibition
HP	highly pathogenic
i.n.	intranasal
LAIV	live attenuated influenza vaccine
MDCK	Madin-Darby canine kidney
MDV	master donor virus
MN	microneutralization
p.i.	post infection
WHO	World Health Organization
NI	neuraminidase-inhibiting

Author details

Yulia Desheva[1,2*]

*Address all correspondence to: desheva@mail.ru

1 Virology Department, Federal State Budgetary Scientific Institution, "Institute of Experimental Medicine", Saint Petersburg, Russian Federation

2 Department of Fundamental Problems of Medicine and Medical Technologies, Saint Petersburg State University, Saint Petersburg, Russian Federation

References

[1] Runstadler J, Hill N, Hussein I, Puryear W, Keogh M. Connecting the study of wild influenza with the potential for pandemic disease. Infection, Genetics and Evolution. 2013;**17**:162-187. DOI: 10.1016/j.meegid.2013.02.020

[2] WHO Technical Report. Avian Influenza Portfolio. Collected Risk Assessments, Technical Guidance to Public Health Authorities and Advice to the Generalpublic. Stockholm, June 2006. Available from: https://ecdc.europa.eu/sites/portal/files/media/en/publications/Publications/0606_TER_Avian_Influenza_Portafolio.pdf [Accessed: Jan 20, 2015]

[3] Rudenko L, Slepushkin A, Monto A, Kendal A, Grigorieva E, Burtseva E, et al. Efficacy of live attenuated and inactivated influenza vaccines in schoolchildren and their unvaccinated contacts in Novgorod, Russia. Journal of Infectious Diseases. 1993;**168**(4):881-887. DOI: 10.1093/infdis/168.4.881

[4] Rudenko L, Lonskaya N, Klimov A, Vasilieva R, Ramirez A. Clinical and epidemiological evaluation of a live, cold-adapted influenza vaccine for 3-14-year-olds. Bulletin of the World Health Organization. 1996;**74**(1):77-84. PMC: 2486837

[5] Rudenko L, Arden N, Grigorieva E, Naychin A, Rekstin A, Klimov A, et al. Immunogenicity and efficacy of Russian live attenuated and US inactivated influenza vaccines used alone and in combination in nursing home residents. Vaccine. 2000;**19**(2-3):308-318. DOI: 10.1016/S0264-410X(00)00153-5

[6] Ambrose C, Luke C, Coelingh K. Current status of live attenuated influenza vaccine in the United States for seasonal and pandemic influenza. Influenza and Other Respiratory Viruses. 2008;**2**(6):193-202. DOI: 10.1111/j.1750-2659.2008.00056.x

[7] WHO Global Action Plan to Increase Vaccine Supply for Influenza Vaccines. Geneva, Belgium. 2006. WHO/IVB/06.13. WHO/ODS/EPR/GIP/2006.1. Available from: (http://whqlibdoc.who.int/hq/2006/WHO IVB 06.13 eng.pdf) [Accessed: Jan 20, 2015]

[8] Cox R, Brokstad K, Ogra P. Influenza virus: Immunity and vaccination strategies. Comparison of the immune response to inactivated and live, attenuated influenza vaccines. Scandinavian Journal of Immunology. 2004;**59**(1):1-15. DOI: 10.1111/j.0300-9475.2004.01382.x

[9] Webster R, Yakhno M, Hinshaw V, Bean W, Copal Murti K. Intestinal influenza: Replication and characterization of influenza viruses in ducks. Virology. 1978;**84**(2):268-278. DOI: 10.1016/0042-6822(78)90247-7

[10] Garcia M, Crawford J, Latimer J, Rivera-Cruz E, Perdue M. Heterogeneity in the haemagglutinin gene and emergence of the highly pathogenic phenotype among recent H5N2 avian influenza viruses from Mexico. Journal of General Virology. 1996;**77**(7):1493-1504. DOI: 10.1099/0022-1317-77-7-1493

[11] Kawaoka Y, Webster R. Evolution of the a/chicken/Pennsylvania/83 (H5N2) influenza virus. Virology. 1985;**146**(1):130-137. DOI: 10.1016/0042-6822(85)90059-5

[12] Selleck P, Arzey G, Kirkland P, Reece R, Gould A, Daniels P, et al. An outbreak of highly pathogenic avian influenza in Australia in 1997 caused by an H7N4 virus. Avian Diseases. 2003;**47**(s3):806-811

[13] Webster RG, Bean WJ, Gorman OT, Chambers TM, Kawaoka Y. Evolution and ecology of influenza A viruses. Microbiological Reviews. 1992;**56**(1):152-179. PMID: 1579108

[14] Becker W. The isolation and classification of tern virus: Influenza virus a/tern/South Africa/1961. Journal of Hygiene. 1966;**64**(03):309-320. DOI: 10.1017/S0022172400040596

[15] Bridges C, Katz J, Seto W, Chan P, Tsang D, Ho W, et al. Risk of influenza A (H5N1) infection among health care workers exposed to patients with influenza A (H5N1), Hong Kong. The Journal of Infectious Diseases. 2000;**181**(1):344-348. DOI: 10.1086/315213

[16] Subbarao K, Klimov A, Katz J, Regnery H, Lim W, Hall H, et al. Characterization of an avian influenza A (H5N1) virus isolated from a child with a fatal respiratory illness. Science. 1998;**279**(5349):393-396. DOI: 10.1126/science.279.5349.393

[17] Claas E, Osterhaus A, van Beek R, De Jong J, Rimmelzwaan G, Senne D, et al. Human influenza A H5N1 virus related to a highly pathogenic avian influenza virus. The Lancet. 1998;**351**(9101):472-477. DOI: 10.1016/S0140-6736(97)11212-0

[18] Hoffmann E, Stech J, Leneva I, Krauss S, Scholtissek C, Chin P, et al. Characterization of the influenza A virus gene pool in avian species in southern China: Was H6N1 a derivative or a precursor of H5N1? Journal of Virology. 2000;**74**(14):6309-6315. DOI: 10.1128/JVI.74.14.6309-6315.2000

[19] Guan Y, Shortridge K, Krauss S, Webster R. Molecular characterization of H9N2 influenza viruses: Were they the donors of the "internal" genes of H5N1 viruses in Hong Kong? Proceedings of the National Academy of Sciences. 1999;**96**(16):9363-9367. DOI: doi.org/10.1073/pnas.96.16.9363

[20] Taubenberger J, Kash J. Influenza virus evolution, host adaptation, and pandemic formation. Cell Host & Microbe. 2010;**7**(6):440-451. DOI: 10.1016/j.chom.2010.05.009

[21] Horimoto T, Fukuda N, Iwatsuki-Horimoto K, Guan Y, Lim W, Peiris M, et al. Antigenic differences between H5N1 human influenza viruses isolated in 1997 and 2003. Journal of Veterinary Medical Science. 2004;**66**(3):303-305. DOI: 10.1292/jvms.66.303

[22] Chen H, Smith G, Li K, Wang J, Fan X, Rayner J, et al. Establishment of multiple sublineages of H5N1 influenza virus in Asia: Implications for pandemic control. Proceedings of the National Academy of Sciences. 2006;**103**(8):2845-2850. DOI: 10.1073/pnas.0511120103

[23] Claes F, Morzaria S, Donis R. Emergence and dissemination of clade 2.3.4.4 H5Nx influenza viruses — How is the Asian HPAI H5 lineage maintained. Current Opinion in Virology. 2016;**16**:158-163. DOI: 10.1016/j.coviro.2016.02.005

[24] Beigel JH, Farrar J, Han AM, Hayden FG, Hyer R, de Jong MD, et al. Avian influenza A (H5N1) infection in humans. The New England Journal of Medicine. 2005;**353**(13):1374-1385. DOI: 10.1056/NEJMra052211

[25] Cumulative Number of Confirmed Human Cases of Avian Influenza A (H5N1) Reported to WHO. May 16, 2017. DOI: 10.3201/eid1107.050070. Available from: http://www.who.int/influenza/human_animal_interface/H5N1_cumulative_table_archives/en/

[26] Schultsz C, Dong V, Chau N, Le N, Lim W, Thanh T, et al. Avian influenza H5N1 and healthcare workers. Emerging Infectious Diseases. 2005;**11**(7):1158-1159. DOI: 10.3201/eid1107.050070

[27] Wang H, Feng Z, Shu Y, Yu H, Zhou L, Zu R, et al. Probable limited person-to-person transmission of highly pathogenic avian influenza A (H5N1) virus in China. The Lancet. 2008;**371**(9622):1427-1434

[28] WHO. Avian Influenza A (H7N9) Virus. Available from: http://www.who.int/influenza/human_animal_interface/influenza_h7n9/en/

[29] Xiang D, Shen X, Pu Z, Irwin DM, Liao M, Shen Y. Convergent evolution of human-isolated H7N9 avian influenza A viruses. The Journal of Infectious Diseases. 2018. DOI: 10.1093/infdis/jiy082

[30] Matrosovich M, Krauss S, Webster R. H9N2 influenza A viruses from poultry in Asia have human virus-like receptor specificity. Virology. 2001;**281**(2):156-162. DOI: 10.1006/viro.2000.0799

[31] Wang M, Fu C, Zheng B. Antibodies against H5 and H9 avian influenza among poultry Workers in China. New England Journal of Medicine. 2009;**360**(24):2583-2584. DOI: 10.1056/NEJMc0900358

[32] Peiris M, Yuen K, Leung C, Chan K, Ip P, Lai R, et al. Human infection with influenza H9N2. The Lancet. 1999;**354**(9182):916-917. DOI: 10.1016/S0140-6736(99)03311-5

[33] Saito T, Lim W, Suzuki T, Suzuki Y, Kida H, Nishimura S, et al. Characterization of a human H9N2 influenza virus isolated in Hong Kong. Vaccine. 2001;**20**(1-2):125-133. DOI: 10.1016/S0264-410X(01)00279-1

[34] Li C, Yu K, Tian G, Yu D, Liu L, Jing B, et al. Evolution of H9N2 influenza viruses from domestic poultry in mainland China. Virology. 2005;**340**(1):70-83. DOI: 10.1016/j.virol.2005.06.025

[35] Guan Y, Shortridge K, Krauss S, Chin P, Dyrting K, Ellis T, et al. H9N2 influenza viruses possessing H5N1-like internal genomes continue to circulate in poultry in Southeastern China. Journal of Virology. 2000;**74**(20):9372-9380. DOI: 10.1128/JVI.74.20.9372-9380.2000

[36] WHO. Antigenic and genetic characteristics of influenza A (H5N1) and influenza A (H9N2) viruses for development of candidate vaccines viruses for pandemic preparedness – February 2011. Releve epidemiologique hebdomadaire. 2011;**86**(11):93-100. Available from: http://www.who.int/wer/2011/wer8611.pdf

[37] Wei SH, Yang JR, Wu HS, Chang MC, Lin JS, Lin CY, et al. Human infection with avian influenza A H6N1 virus: An epidemiological analysis. The Lancet Respiratory medicine. 2013;**1**(10):771-778. DOI: 10.1016/S2213-2600(13)70221-2

[38] Zhou NN, Senne DA, Landgraf JS, Swenson SL, Erickson G, Rossow K, et al. Genetic reassortment of avian, swine, and human influenza A viruses in American pigs. Journal of Virology 1999;**73**(10):8851-8856. PMID: 10482643

[39] Huang K, Bahl J, Fan X, Vijaykrishna D, Cheung C, Webby R, et al. Establishment of an H6N2 influenza virus lineage in domestic ducks in southern China. Journal of Virology. 2010;**84**(14):6978-6986. DOI: 10.1128/JVI.00256-10

[40] WHO. Antigenic and Genetic Characteristics of Zoonotic Influenza Viruses and Development of Candidate Vaccine Viruses for Pandemic Preparedness. September 2017. Available from: http://www.who.int/influenza/vaccines/virus/201709_zoonotic_vaccinevirusupdate.pdf?ua=1

[41] Li S, Liu C, Klimov A, Subbarao K, Perdue M, Mo D, et al. Recombinant influenza A virus vaccines for the pathogenic human A/Hong Kong/97 (H5N1) viruses. The Journal of Infectious Diseases. 1999;**179**(5):1132-1138. DOI: 10.1086/314713

[42] Horimoto T, Takada A, Fujii K, Goto H, Hatta M, Watanabe S, et al. The development and characterization of H5 influenza virus vaccines derived from a 2003 human isolate. Vaccine. 2006;**24**(17):3669-3676. DOI: 10.1016/j.vaccine.2005.07.005

[43] Suguitan A, McAuliffe J, Mills K, Jin H, Duke G, Lu B, et al. Live, attenuated influenza A H5N1 candidate vaccines provide broad cross-protection in mice and ferrets. PLoS Medicine. 2006;**3**(9):e360. DOI: 10.1371/journal.pmed.0030360

[44] Boonnak K, Matsuoka Y, Wang W, Suguitan A, Chen Z, Paskel M, et al. Development of clade-specific and broadly reactive live attenuated influenza virus vaccines against rapidly evolving H5 subtype viruses. Journal of Virology. 2017;**91**(15):e00547-17. DOI: 10.1128/JVI.00547-17

[45] Joseph T, McAuliffe J, Lu B, Vogel L, Swayne D, Jin H, et al. A live attenuated cold-adapted influenza A H7N3 virus vaccine provides protection against homologous and heterologous H7 viruses in mice and ferrets. Virology. 2008;**378**(1):123-132. DOI: 10.1016/j.virol.2008.05.021

[46] Chen H, Subbarao K, Swayne D, Chen Q, Lu X, Katz J, et al. Generation and evaluation of a high-growth reassortant H9N2 influenza A virus as a pandemic vaccine candidate. Vaccine. 2003;**21**(17-18):1974-1979. DOI: 10.1016/S0264-410X(02)00809-5

[47] Horimoto T, Kawaoka Y. The Hemagglutinin cleavability of a virulent avian influenza virus by Subtilisin-like Endoproteases is influenced by the amino acid immediately downstream of the cleavage site. Virology. 1995;**210**(2):466-470. DOI: 10.1006/viro.1995.1363

[48] Wareing M, Marsh G, Tannock G. Preparation and characterisation of attenuated cold-adapted influenza A reassortants derived from the a/Leningrad/134/17/57 donor strain. Vaccine. 2002;**20**(16):2082-2090. DOI: 10.1016/S0264-410X(02)00056-7

[49] Desheva J, Rudenko L, Alexandrova G, Lu X, Rekstin A, Katz J, et al. Reassortment between avian apathogenic and human attenuated cold-adapted viruses as an approach for preparing influenza pandemic vaccines. International Congress Series. 2004;**1263**:724-727. DOI: 10.1016/j.ics.2004.02.043

[50] Desheva J, Rudenko L, Rekstin A, Swayne D, Cox N, Klimov A. Development of candidate H7N3 live attenuated cold–adapted influenza vaccine. In: Proceedings of the International Conference on Options for the Control of Influenza VI, Toronto, Ontario, Canada. Jun 17-23, 2007. pp. 591-592

[51] Desheva YA, Smolonogina TA, Rudenko LG. A preclinical trial of the reassortant influenza virus vaccine strain a/17/quail/Hong Kong/97/84 (H9N2). Voprosy virusologii. 2015;**60**(4):40-44. PMID: 26665434

[52] Desheva Y, Smolonogina T, Landgraf G, Rudenko L. Development of the a/H6N1 influenza vaccine candidate based on a/Leningrad/134/17/57 (H2N2) master donor virus and the genome composition analysis using high resolution melting (HRM). Microbiology Independent Research journal. 2016;**3**(1):61-67. DOI: 10.18527/2500-2236-2016-3-1-42-48

[53] Subbarao K, Park E, Lawson C, Chen Y, Murphy B. Sequential addition of temperature-sensitive missense mutations into the PB2 gene of influenza A transfectant viruses can effect an increase in temperature sensitivity and attenuation and permits the rational design of a genetically engineered live influenza A virus vaccine. Journal of Virology. 1995;**69**(10):5969-5977. DOI: 10.1016/j.vaccine.2006.06.023

[54] Desheva J, Lu X, Rekstin A, Rudenko L, Swayne D, Cox N, et al. Characterization of an influenza A H5N2 reassortant as a candidate for live-attenuated and inactivated vaccines against highly pathogenic H5N1 viruses with pandemic potential. Vaccine. 2006;**24**(47-48):6859-6866

[55] Lu X, Edwards L, Desheva J, Nguyen D, Rekstin A, Stephenson I, et al. Cross-protective immunity in mice induced by live-attenuated or inactivated vaccines against highly pathogenic influenza A (H5N1) viruses. Vaccine. 2006;**24**(44-46):6588-6593. DOI: 10.1016/j.vaccine.2006.05.039

[56] Desheva Y, Leontieva G, Kramskaya T, Smolonogina T, Grabovskaya K, Landgraf G, et al. Prevention of influenza A (H7N9) and bacterial infections in mice using intranasal immunization with live influenza vaccine and the group B Streptococcus recombinant polypeptides. Virology: Research and Treatment. 2017;**8**:1-10. DOI: 10.1177/1178122X17710949

[57] Rudenko L, Isakova-Sivak I. Pandemic preparedness with live attenuated influenza vaccines based on a/Leningrad/134/17/57 master donor virus. Expert Review of Vaccines. 2015;**14**(3):395-412. DOI: 10.1586/14760584.2015.979159

[58] Matsuda K, Shibata T, Sakoda Y, Kida H, Kimura T, Ochiai K, et al. In vitro demonstration of neural transmission of avian influenza A virus. The Journal of general virology. 2005;**86**(Pt 4):1131-1139. DOI: 10.1099/vir.0.80704-0

[59] Couch R, Kasel J. Immunity to influenza in man. Annual Review of Microbiology. 1983;**37**(1):529-549. DOI: 10.1146/annurev.mi.37.100183.002525

[60] Renegar K, Small P, Boykins L, Wright P. Role of IgA versus IgG in the control of influenza viral infection in the murine respiratory tract. The Journal of Immunology. 2004;**173**(3):1978-1986. DOI: 10.4049/jimmunol.173.3.1978

[61] Mazanec M, Kaetzel C, Lamm M, Fletcher D, Nedrud J. Intracellular neutralization of virus by immunoglobulin a antibodies. Proceedings of the National Academy of Sciences. 1992;**89**(15):6901-6905. PMID: 1323121

[62] Treanor J, Snyder M, London W, Murphy B. The B allele of the NS gene of avian influenza viruses, but not the a allele, attenuates a human influenza A virus for squirrel monkeys. Virology. 1989;**171**(1):1-9. DOI: 10.1016/0042-6822(89)90504-7

[63] Rimmelzwaan G, Kuiken T, van Amerongen G, Bestebroer T, Fouchier R, Osterhaus A. A primate model to study the pathogenesis of influenza A (H5N1) virus infection. Avian Diseases. 2003;**47**(s3):931-933. DOI: 10.1637/0005-2086-47.s3.931

[64] Rudenko L. Live attenuated vaccine in Russia: Advantages, further research and development. In proceedings of the international conference on options for the control of influenza VI, Toronto, Ontario, Canada. Jun 17-23, 2007. pp. 122-124

[65] Rudenko L, Desheva J, Korovkin S, Mironov A, Rekstin A, Grigorieva E, et al. Safety and immunogenicity of live attenuated influenza reassortant H5 vaccine (phase I-II clinical trials). Influenza and Other Respiratory Viruses. 2008;**2**(6):203-209. DOI: 10.1111/j.1750-2659.2008.00064.x

[66] Rudenko L, Kiseleva I, Naykhin A, Erofeeva M, Stukova M, Donina S, et al. Assessment of human immune responses to H7 avian influenza virus of pandemic potential: Results from a placebo–controlled, randomized double–blind phase I study of live attenuated H7N3 influenza vaccine. PLoS One. 2014;**9**(2):e87962. DOI: 10.1371/journal.pone.0087962

[67] Chirkova T, Naykhin A, Petukhova G, Korenkov D, Donina S, Mironov A, et al. Memory T-cell immune response in healthy young adults vaccinated with live attenuated influenza A (H5N2) vaccine. Clinical and Vaccine Immunology. 2011;**18**(10):1710-1718. DOI: 10.1128/CVI.05116-11

[68] Wood J, Nicholson K, Stephenson I, Zambon M, Newman R, Major D, et al. Experience with the clinical development of influenza vaccines for potential pandemics. Medical Microbiology and Immunology. 2002;**191**(3-4):197-201. DOI: 10.1007/s00430-002-0146-x

[69] Rudenko L, Isakova-Sivak I, Rekstin A. H7N9: Can H7N3 live-attenuated influenza vaccine be used at the early stage of the pandemic? Expert Review of Vaccines. 2013;**13**(1): 1-4. DOI: 10.1586/14760584.2014.864564

[70] Memoli M, Shaw P, Han A, Czajkowski L, Reed S, Athota R, et al. Evaluation of anti-hemagglutinin and antineuraminidase antibodies as correlates of protection in an influenza A/H1N1 virus healthy human challenge model. MBio Journal. 2016;**7**(2):e00417-16. DOI: 10.1128/mBio.00417-16

[71] Smolonogina TA, Desheva Iu A, Rekstin AR, Mironov AN, Rudenko LG. [Evaluation of the anti-neuraminidase antibodies in clinical trials of the live influenza vaccine of the a(H5N2) subtype]. Voprosy virusologii. 2013;**58**(6):31-35. PMID: 24772644

Section 5

Impact of Adjuvants on Influenza Vaccines

Chapter 5

The Impact of Adjuvanted and Non-Adjuvanted Influenza Vaccines on the Innate and Adaptive Immunity Effectors

Mikhail Petrovich Kostinov,
Nelli Kimovna Akhmatova,
Ekaterina Alexandrovna Khromova,
Svetlana Anatolyevna Skhodova,
Vera Nikolaevna Stolpnikova,
Alexander Petrovich Cherdantsev and
Anna Egorovna Vlasenko

Additional information is available at the end of the chapter

http://dx.doi.org/10.5772/intechopen.77006

Abstract

To date, the advantage of adjuvanted over non-adjuvanted vaccines in the specific antibodies formation is proved. However, cellular mechanisms, including parameters of the innate immunity, involved in the vaccine-induced immune response are not well studied. The human study of inactivated vaccines showed that both subunit vaccine and split vaccine induced cellular immune response, but adjuvanted vaccine containing Polyoxidonium had the greatest potential. Despite the fact that influenza vaccines must activate endosomal receptors, they cause non-specific activation of the surface TLRs. They can trigger intracellular signals leading to the induction of antiviral mechanisms and to the activation of the body's protective resources against microbial infections. To assess the immunological efficacy of adjuvanted vaccines and humoral reactions to vaccination it is necessary to evaluate activation of cellular mechanisms of innate and adaptive immunity.

Keywords: influenza vaccines, adjuvanted influenza vaccine, lymphocyte subpopulations, toll-like receptors

1. Introduction

Vaccination is the most effective means of preventing influenza and consequently reducing incidence and severity of complications. Modern influenza vaccines include a live attenuated, inactivated (whole-virion, split-virion and subunit) vaccines. Currently, inactivated split and subunit vaccines are used for influenza prevention as the safest ones and stimulating the production of a protective level of strain-specific virus-neutralizing antibodies to the globular domain of hemagglutinin protein and neuraminidase protein of contemporary serotypes of the influenza virus. These vaccines protect against infection with the appropriate antigenic variants of influenza virus. Not all inactivated vaccines have been reported to be effective enough for certain categories of vaccinated people [1–7]. Some of them are not able to protect against drift variants of influenza virus [8–11].

Due to the continuous antigenic drift of influenza viruses and the emergence of pandemic influenza viruses, the study of influenza vaccines causing broader protective immunity is of great interest [12]. In this regard, before influenza pandemic of 2009–2010 vaccination with adjuvanted vaccines began, aiming to enhance the synthesis of specific antibodies. In addition, given poor population health in the modern era, there is the need to enhance the efficacy of vaccines meant to activate all the components of the immune system. According to the literature data, adjuvanted vaccines seem to have such effect. However, a small number of human studies to investigate, how adjuvanted vaccine influence cellular immunity and activate of not only adaptive, but also innate immunity, have been conducted. In addition, unlike foreign adjuvanted influenza vaccines developed in 2009–2010, the National Immunization Calendar of the Russian Federation for more than 20 years applies polymer-subunit influenza vaccine containing immunomodulator PO as the adjuvant. Furthermore, immunomodulators have long been used in vaccination practice for immunocompromised patients in the Russian Federation. Immunomodulator use to support the vaccination was shown to promptly enhance the synthesis of specific antibodies and significantly decrease the incidence of respiratory infections in the postvaccinal period [13–15].

To date, the vaccine immunogenicity is assessed according to the requirements of the European Committee for influenza vaccines [16], and must meet at least one of the three criteria:

- seroconversion (percentage of subjects with a fourfold increase in antibody titers after vaccination)—at least 40%;
- seroprotection (percentage of subjects with a protective antibody titers before and 21–28 days after vaccination)—at least 70% and
- multiplicity factor for the increase of antibody titers compared to baseline—at least 2.5.

Taking into account a new type of vaccine (adjuvanted), not only humoral, but also cellular immune response is important for the evaluation of immunological efficacy. The activation of cellular immunity parameters, important to the formation of immunological memory, may differ from that of non-adjuvanted vaccines.

The aim of the study was to examine the effect of immunoadjuvant-containing and non-adjuvanted influenza vaccines on the immunophenotype of healthy donor lymphocytes and the number of cells with toll-like receptor expression *in vitro*.

2. Materials and methods

2.1. Clinical characteristics of patients

An open-label non-randomized monocenter study enrolled 27 healthy women of childbearing potential (aged 18–40 years) without co-morbidities who were not influenza-vaccinated within the previous 3 years and acquired no influenza or influenza-like illnesses within the previous 6 months.

2.2. Legal basis of the study

Once the signed informed consent for study participation was obtained, venous blood samples were drawn from volunteers with all applied aseptic and antiseptic techniques met and in accordance with the Study Protocol approved in 2015 by the Ethics Committee at the Mechnikov Research Institute of Vaccines and Sera. The study was conducted at the certified laboratory of the Mechnikov Research Institute of Vaccines and Sera (Moscow) using modern reagents and equipment.

2.3. Distribution pattern of lymphocyte subpopulations

The distribution pattern of peripheral blood lymphocyte subpopulations *in vitro* in healthy women exposed to influenza vaccine was tested by flow cytometer FC-500 (Beckman Coulter, USA), using anti-CD45/CD3, anti-CD45/CD3/CD4, anti-CD45/CD3/CD8, anti-CD16/56, anti-CD3/CD16/56, anti-CD45/CD20, anti-CD8/HLA-DR, anti-CD3/HLA-DR, anti-CD45/CD25, and anti-CD4/CD25/Foxp3 FITC- and PE-labeled monoclonal antibodies mAbs (Beckman Coulter, USA).

2.4. Toll-like receptors

The concentration of granulocytes with TLR expression was evaluated by flow cytometer FC-500 (Beckman Coulter, USA) using anti-TLR2, anti-TLR 3, anti-TLR4, anti-TLR6, anti-TLR8, and anti-TLR9 mAbs (eBioscience, USA).

Mononuclear WBCs were isolated from the whole blood using Ficoll-Urografin density gradients. We incubated 10^6 cells/mL in RPMI-1640 complete growth medium (PanEco, Russia) with 10% FBS (PanEco, Russia) and antibiotic (streptomycin) in the presence of 10 μL of a corresponding vaccine for 72 hours.

2.5. Study vaccines

Influvac ("Abbott biologicals" B.V., Netherlands) – inactivated subunit influenza vaccine, Vaxigrip ("Sanofi Pasteur", France)– inactivated split-virion influenza vaccine for influenza prevention. These vaccines contain hemagglutinin of the influenza virus type A subtypes A/H1N1 и A/H3N2 (15 μg each) and hemagglutinin of the influenza virus type B (15 μg). Grippol plus (LLC "NPO Petrovax Pharm," Russia) – trivalent polymer subunit inactivated influenza vaccine. It contains hemagglutinin of the influenza virus type A subtypes A/H1N1 и A/H3N2 and hemagglutinin of the influenza virus type B (5 μg each), and immunoadjuvant Polyoxidonium (500 μg). All the vaccines contained current influenza virus strains for epidemiological seasons 2015–2016 and 2016–2017.

Anti-influenza virus A/H1N1/California/07/09, p.149, A/H3N2/Switzerland/9715293/13 (subunit antigen), B/Phuket/3073/13, p. 25 (season 2015–2016); A/H1N1/California/07/09 p.124 till 01.17, A/H3N2/Hong Kong/4801/14 p.200, and B/Brisbane/60/08 p. 27 (season 2016–2017) **baseline serum antibody levels** were studied in volunteers using the standard method (MU 3.3.2 1758–03) for HAI assay. The 4+ system was applied to HAI assay: an antigen titer, i.e., 1 HAU, was highest antigen dilution giving complete hemagglutination of RBCs (3+ or 4+). In HAI assay the antigen working dose was the antigen dilution containing 4 hemagglutination units (4 HAU) in 0.2 mL.

2.6. Statistical analysis

Cell percentage difference between test groups was measured by a robust dispersion analysis of repeated measures (R Statistical Software, WRS2 package, rmanova function) with subsequent pairwise comparisons (R Statistical Software, WRS2 package, rmmcp function), the obtained significance level was corrected by Holm method [17]. Benjamini-Hochberg method was used to account for multiple comparison (false discovery rate control) [18]. The obtained data were described with the median and interquartile range.

3. Study results

First, we estimated vaccine effect on distribution pattern of lymphocyte subpopulations in PBMC cultures. Volunteers were divided into three groups according to the baseline antibody (AB) titers against the hemagglutin of the influenza virus A/H1N1, A/H3N2, and B: low AB titers (20–40 U) in the first group, medium AB titers (80–160 U) in the second group, and high AB titers (≥320 U) in the third group. Such differences in AB level indicate that influenza infection in the unvaccinated volunteers could have been masked under the guise of another infection, as all volunteers did not report previous influenza infection.

Immunophenotypic analysis showed changes in the number of T lymphocytes (CD45+/CD3+), NK cells (CD16+/56+), NKT cells (CD3 + CD16/56+), B lymphocytes (CD45+/CD20+), and activated cells (**Table 1**).

There were statistically significant differences ($F = 8.00$, $p < 0.001$, $q = 0.001$) in T lymphocytes (CD3+) distribution after incubation with different types of vaccines (**Figure 1**). It should be noted that regardless of the AB level vaccines did not have a significant effect on T lymphocyte number except subunit vaccine, which caused a decrease in the percent of T lymphocytes compared to control (PBMC culture without vaccine) while the absolute number did not change. These results may indicate a shift in the number of cells due to an increase in the number of other subpopulations.

Lymphocyte subpopulations	N	% in comparison groups – Me(Q1–Q3)				F	p	q
		Control	Subunit V	Adjuvanted V	Split-product V			
T lymphocytes (CD45/CD3+)	18	79.85 (74.17–83.35)	71.25 (64.7–79.75)	74.6 (66.38–79.17)	73.91 (66.92–78.22)	8.00	<0.001	0.001
Helper T cells (CD45/CD3/CD4+)	21	43.5 (41–49.8)	37.5 (32.7–43.8)	40.2 (31.8–46.5)	41.9 (35.6–47.7)	2.50	0.071	0.107
Cytotoxic T lymphocytes, CTL (CD45/CD3/CD8+)	21	23.5 (17.3–24.7)	21.2 (17.4–23.6)	22.5 (16.9–26.9)	21.5 (18.4–5.8)	0.64	0.533	0.601
Natural killer cells, NK cells (CD16/56+)	24	4.85 (4.175–5.9)	13.2 (11.15–14.85)	17.25 (15.93–18.25)	15 (13.8–16.25)	180.28	<0.001	<0.001
Natural killer T cells, NKT (CD3/CD16/56+)	24	1.6 (1.3–2.25)	3.6 (2.775–5.825)	7.5 (6.675–8.225)	5 (4.625–6.75)	57.52	<0.001	0.00001
B lymphocytes (CD45/CD20+)	24	5.15 (4.475–6.725)	16.36 (15.47–17.7)	21.15 (18.93–22.9)	18.1 (15.88–19.62)	167.44	<0.001	<0.001
Activated cytotoxic T lymphocytes, CTL(CD8/HLA-DR+)	20	0.4 (0.275–0.5)	0.7 (0.3–1.2)	1.6 (1.2–2.4)	1.35 (0.4875–1.975)	13.36	<0.001	<0.001
Activated T lymphocytes (CD3/HLA-DR+)	12	1.05 (0.65–1.65)	2.7 (1.875–3.375)	4.95 (3.775–7.1)	2.6 (1.9–3.575)	8.92	<0.001	0.002
Activated lymphocytes (CD45/CD25+)	16	1.45 (1–1.775)	3.7 (2.6–4.85)	4.15 (3.2–9.075)	4.15 (3.075–5.275)	12.94	<0.001	0.001
Regulatory T cells, Tregs (CD4/CD25/Foxp3+)	13	2.7 (1.7–2.9)	3.5 (3.2–4.9)	3.7 (3.2–5.5)	4.2 (2.2–4.5)	4.27	0.017	0.032
IRI (CD4/CD8)	20	1.825 (1.5–3.275)	1.85 (1.45–2.325)	1.85 (1.4–2.5)	1.65 (1.475–.525)	1.26	0.300	0.389

Note. Aliquots of 10 μL vaccines were added to cell suspensions (PBMC, 10^6 cells/mL). Cells were incubated for 72 hours at 37°C in 5% CO_2. The cells were then washed with RPMI-1640 at 1500 g for 10 min. Monoclonal antibodies against studied cell receptors were added in accordance with the manufacturer's instructions. The number of cells (%) in each sample was determined by flow cytometry.

Table 1. Distribution pattern of peripheral blood lymphocyte subpopulations incubated with influenza vaccines.

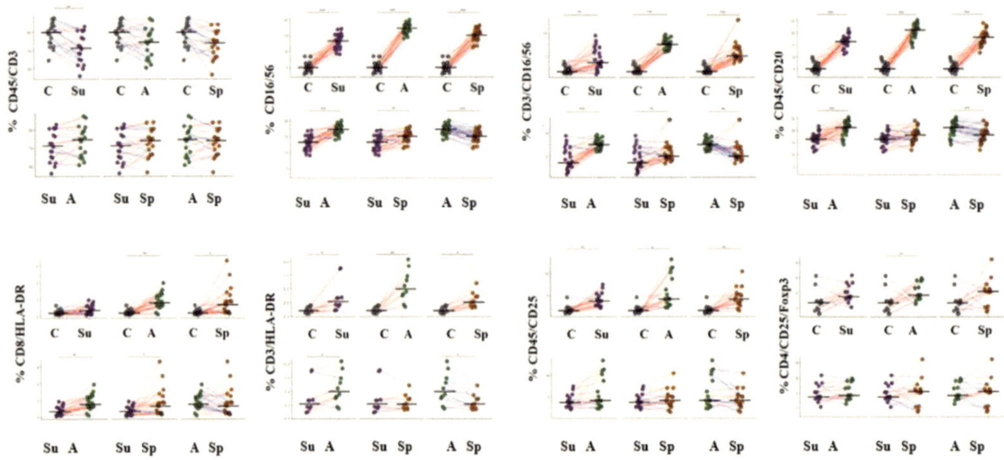

Figure 1. Lymphocyte count in PBMC culture after incubation with influenza vaccines. C = control; Su = inactivated subunit influenza vaccine; A = trivalent inactivated polymer-subunit influenza vaccine; Sp = inactivated split-product influenza vaccine.

The comparison of the T lymphocyte count between vaccines showed a significant decrease in the number of cells after incubation with subunit vaccine only (71.2% vs. 79.8% in control, $p = 0.008$) (**Figure 1**). However, the changes in the T lymphocyte (CD3+) number after incubation with different types of vaccines were observed only in women with medium AB level ($F = 6.40$, $p = 0.004$, $q = 0.007$). In this group, statistically significant differences were found for subunit vaccine (72 vs. 82.6% in control, $p = 0.022$) and split-product vaccine (74.8 vs. 82.6% in control, $p = 0.022$) (**Figure 2**).

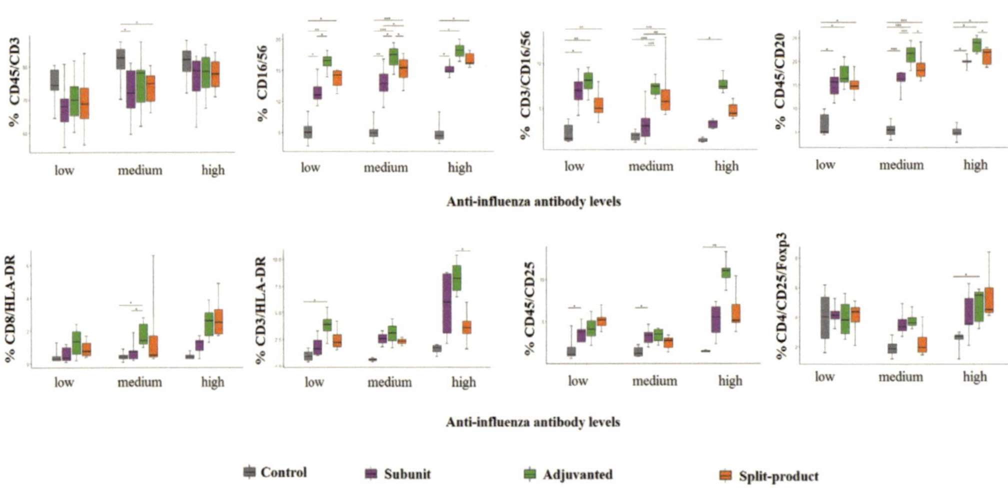

Figure 2. The impact of influenza vaccines on the lymphocyte count in PBMC cultures from volunteers with different antibody titers against the hemagglutinin of the influenza virus a/H1N1, a/H3N2, and B. Significant differences: *** $p < 0.001$, ** $p < 0.01$, * $p < 0.05$.

Analysis revealed significant changes ($F = 180.28$, $p < 0.001$, $q < 0.001$) in percent of natural killer cells (NK, CD16/56+) after incubation with different types of vaccines (**Table 1**, **Figure 1**). Regardless of the AB level there was an increase in number of NK cells from 4.8 (control) to 13.2% (subunit vaccine), 17.2% (adjuvanted vaccine), and 15% (split vaccine). There were statistically significant differences for subunit (13.2 vs. 4.8%, $p < 0.001$), adjuvanted (17.2 vs. 4.8%, $p < 0.001$), and split vaccines (15 vs. 4.8%, $p < 0.001$) compared to control, for subunit vaccine compared to adjuvanted (13.2% vs. 17.2%, $p < 0.001$) and split vaccines (13.2 vs. 15%, $p = 0.003$), and for adjuvanted vaccine compared to split vaccine (17.2 vs. 15%, $p < 0.001$). That means that incubation with influenza vaccines increased the number of NK cells in all cultures.

However, the changes in number of NK cells (CD16/56+) after incubation of PBMC with different types of vaccines were observed in all groups of volunteers, regardless of the baseline anti-influenza AB level ($F = 48.88$, $p < 0.001$, $q < 0.001$ – low AB level, $F = 103.04$, $p < 0.001$, $q < 0.001$ – medium AB level, $F = 89.09$, $p < 0.001$, $q < 0.001$ – high AB level) (**Figure 2**).In women with low anti-influenza AB level, percent of NK cells (CD16/56+) was significantly higher after incubation with subunit (11 vs. 5%, $p = 0.045$), adjuvanted (16.5% vs. 5%, $p = 0.001$), and split vaccines (14.2 vs. 5%, $p = 0.01$) compared to control. Immunoadjuvant-containing vaccine had a higher potential for elevation of NK cell number (3.3-fold increase) compared with subunit vaccine (2.2-fold increase) ($p = 0.017$).

In women with medium anti-influenza AB level, percent of NK cells (CD16/56+) was significantly higher after incubation with subunit (12.8 vs. 4.8%, $p = 0.001$), adjuvanted (17.5 vs. 4.8%, $p < 0.001$), and split vaccines (15.3 vs. 4.8%, $p < 0.001$) compared to control. This corresponds to a 2.6- to 3.6-fold increase. Immunoadjuvant-containing vaccine produced more pronounced increase compared to subunit vaccine (17.5 vs. 12.8%, $p = 0.029$) and split vaccine (17.5 vs. 15.3%, $p = 0.011$), and number of NK cells was significantly higher after incubation with split vaccine compared to subunit vaccine (15.3 vs.12.8%, $p = 0.029$).

In women with high anti-influenza AB level, percent of NK cells (CD16/56+) was significantly higher after incubation with subunit (14.8 vs. 4.4%, $p = 0.023$), adjuvanted (18.2 vs. 4.4%, $p = 0.046$), and split vaccines (16.1 vs. 4.4%, $p = 0.035$) compared to control. This corresponds to a 3.3-, 4.1-, and 3.6-fold increase, respectively. There were no statistically significant differences between various types of vaccines.

For NKT cells (natural killer T cells, CD3 + CD16/56+), following findings were revealed. Regardless of the AB level there were statistically significant changes ($F = 57.52$, $p < 0.001$, $q < 0.001$) in NKT cells distribution after incubation with different types of vaccines: for subunit (3.6 vs. 1.6%, $p = 0.006$), adjuvanted (7.5 vs. 1.6%, $p < 0.001$), and split vaccines (5 vs. 1.6%, $p < 0.001$) compared to control, for subunit vaccine compared to adjuvanted (3.6 vs. 7.5%, $p < 0.001$) and split vaccines (3.6 vs. 5%, $p = 0.007$), and for adjuvanted vaccine compared to split vaccine (7.5 vs. 5%, $p = 0.006$). Therefore, subunit vaccine caused a 2.2-fold increase in NKT cell number, adjuvanted vaccine caused a 4.6-fold increase, and split vaccine caused a 3.1-fold increase compared to control (**Table 1**, **Figure 1**).

An increase of NKT cell (CD3 + CD16/56+) number in all cultures was dependent of baseline anti-influenza AB level ($F = 22.08$, $p < 0.001$, $q < 0.001$ – low AB level, $F = 20.02$, $p < 0.001$, $q < 0.001$ – medium AB level, $F = 65.92$, $p < 0.001$, $q < 0.001$ – high AB level) (**Figure 2**).

In women with low anti-influenza AB level, NKT cell (CD16/56+) number was significantly higher after *in vitro* incubation with subunit (7 vs. 1.6%, p = 0.033), adjuvanted (8.1 vs. 1.6%, p = 0.007), and split vaccines (5 vs. 1.6%, p = 0.005) compared to control. There were no statistically significant differences between various types of vaccines.

In women with medium anti-influenza AB level, NKT cell number in PBMC cultures was significantly higher after incubation with adjuvanted vaccine compared to control (7.4 vs. 1.3%, p < 0.001) and subunit vaccine (7.4 vs. 3%, p < 0.001) (5.7- and 2.48-fold increase, respectively) and after incubation with split vaccine compared to control (4.4 vs. 1.3%, p < 0.001) and subunit vaccine (4.4 vs. 3%, p = 0.009) (3.38- and 1.46-fold increase, respectively).

In women with high anti-influenza AB level, percent of NKT cells (CD3 + CD16/56+) was significantly (4.6-fold) higher after incubation with adjuvanted vaccine compared to control (7.4 vs. 1.6%, p = 0.043).

Analysis also revealed statistically significant differences (F = 167.44, p < 0.001, q < 0.001) in B lymphocytes (CD45/CD20+) distribution after incubation of PBMC with different types of vaccines (regardless of the AB level): for subunit (16.3 vs. 5.1%, 3.1-fold increase, p < 0.001), adjuvanted (21.1 vs. 5.1%, 4.1-fold increase, p < 0.001), and split vaccines (18.1 vs. 5.1%, 3.5-fold increase, p < 0.001) compared to control, and for adjuvanted vaccine compared to subunit (21.1 vs. 16.3%, 1.3-fold increase, p < 0.001) and split vaccines (21.1 vs. 18.1%, 1.1-fold increase, p < 0.001). Therefore, adjuvanted vaccine was the most effective (**Table 1**, **Figure 1**).

Regardless of the AB level there was a significant increase in B lymphocyte number after incubation with different types of vaccines (F = 24.09, p < 0.001, q < 0.001 – low AB level, F = 181.14, p < 0.001, q < 0.001 – medium AB level, F = 150.61, p < 0.001, q < 0.001 – high AB level) (**Figure 2**). In women with low anti-influenza AB level, percent of B lymphocytes (CD20+) was significantly higher after incubation with subunit (15.6 vs. 5%, p = 0.017), adjuvanted (16.3 vs. 5%, p = 0.046), and split vaccines (14.7 vs. 5%, p = 0.014) compared to control. There were no statistically significant differences between various types of vaccines.

In women with medium anti-influenza AB level, percent of B lymphocytes (CD20+) was also significantly higher after incubation with all types of vaccines: subunit (16.2 vs. 5.3%, p < 0.001), adjuvanted (21.6 vs. 5.3%, p < 0.001), and split vaccines (18.1 vs. 5.3%, p < 0.001) compared to control. Immunoadjuvant-containing vaccine had the greatest potential for elevation of B lymphocyte number (21.6%) compared with subunit vaccine (16.2%, 1.3-fold increase) (p < 0.001) and split vaccine (18.1%, 1.2-fold increase) (p = 0.013).

In women with high anti-influenza AB level, there was a significant increase in B lymphocyte number after incubation with subunit (20 vs. 4.7%, p = 0.021), adjuvanted (23.6 vs. 4.7%, p = 0.030), and split vaccines (21.9 vs. 4.7%, p = 0.030) compared to control. Immunoadjuvant-containing vaccine induced higher (fivefold) increase of B lymphocyte number than split vaccine (4.6-fold, p = 0.011).

Analysis revealed statistically significant differences (F = 13.36, p < 0.001, q < 0.001) in the distribution of activated cytotoxic T lymphocytes (CD8/HLA-DR+) after incubation of PBMC with different types of vaccines (regardless of the AB level) (**Table 1**, **Figure 1**).

Immunoadjuvant-containing and split vaccines more effectively increased the number of this type of cells. There were statistically significant changes for subunit (1.6 vs. 0.4%, $p < 0.001$), adjuvanted (1.3 vs. 0.4%, $p = 0.050$), and split vaccines (1.6 vs. 0.7%, $p = 0.002$) compared to control, for adjuvanted vaccine compared to subunit vaccine (1.3 vs. 0.7%, respectively, $p = 0.046$), and for adjuvanted vaccine compared to split vaccine (4.9 vs. 2.6%, respectively, $p = 0.044$).

However, changes in the number of activated cytotoxic T lymphocytes *in vitro* between vaccine types were significant only in women with medium anti-influenza AB level ($F = 5.16$, $p = 0.020$, $q = 0.035$) (**Figure 2**). Incubation with adjuvanted vaccine caused significant increase of the number of activated cytotoxic T lymphocytes compared to control (1.4 vs. 0.4%, $p = 0.049$) and subunit vaccine (1.4 vs. 0.7%, $p = 0.047$).

Regardless of the AB level there were significant changes in the number of T lymphocytes with late activation marker (CD3/HLA-DR+) after incubation with different types of vaccines ($F = 8.92$, $p < 0.001$, $q = 0.002$) (**Table 1**, **Figure 1**). There were statistically significant changes for subunit (2.7 vs. 1%, $p < 0.044$), adjuvanted (4.9 vs. 1%, $p = 0.006$), and split vaccines (2.6 vs. 1%, $p = 0.010$) compared to control, and for adjuvanted vaccine compared to subunit (4.9 vs. 2.7%, $p = 0.015$) and split vaccines (4.9 vs. 2.6%, $p = 0.044$).

Statistically significant changes in the number of this type of cells were demonstrated only in women with low ($F = 30.17$, $p < 0.001$, $q < 0.001$) and high ($F = 12.49$, $p = 0.001$, $q = 0.003$) anti-influenza AB level (**Figure 2**). In women with low serum AB level, analysis of activated T lymphocytes showed significant activation by adjuvanted vaccine compared to control (3.8 vs. 0.9%, $p = 0.047$). In women with high serum AB level, the number of activated T lymphocytes was significantly higher after incubation with adjuvanted vaccine compared to split vaccine (8.2 vs. 3.5%, $p = 0.027$) (**Figure 2**).

For lymphocytes with early activation marker (CD45/CD25+), there was statistically significant increase ($F = 12.94$, $p < 0.001$, $q = 0.001$) after incubation of PBMC with different types of vaccines, regardless of the AB level (**Table 1**, **Figure 1**).All types of vaccines increased number of cells with early activation marker. Furthermore, there were statistically significant changes for subunit (3.7 vs. 1.4%, $p = 0.007$), adjuvanted (4.1 vs. 1.45%, $p = 0.049$), and split-product vaccines (4.1 vs. 1.4%, $p = 0.003$) compared to control. There were no statistically significant differences between various types of vaccines.

Regardless of the AB level there was a significant changes in the number of activated CD45/CD25+ lymphocytes. It was dependent of the vaccine type in all groups of volunteers ($F = 9.96$, $p = 0.002$, $q = 0.006$ – low AB level, $F = 7.92$, $p = 0.002$, $q = 0.005$ – medium AB level, $F = 25.89$, $p < 0.001$, $q < 0.001$ – high AB level) (**Figure 2**).

In women with low and medium AB level, percent of T lymphocytes with early activation marker (CD45/CD25+) was significantly increased after incubation of PBMC with subunit vaccine (3.8 and 3.3%, respectively) compared to control (1.1 and 1.2%, respectively) ($p = 0.024$ and $p = 0.036$). At the same time, in women with high AB level, the number of these cells was increased after incubation of PBMC with adjuvanted vaccine (11%) compared to control (1.5%) ($p = 0.009$).

Analysis also revealed significant changes (F = 4.27, p = 0.017, q = 0.032) in regulatory T cell (T-regs) number with CD4/CD25/Foxp3+ phenotype after incubation of PBMC with different types of vaccines, regardless of the AB level (**Table 1**, **Figure 1**). Immunoadjuvant-containing vaccine increased T-regs number compared to control (3.7 vs. 2.7%, 1.3-fold increase, p = 0.005). Other types of vaccines did not have a significant effect on these cells.

Significant changes in the number of T-regs between vaccine types were noted only in women with high AB level against influenza viruses A/H1N1, A/H3N2, and B (F = 8.15, p = 0.003, q = 0.006) (**Figure 2**).Incubation of PBMC with adjuvanted vaccine induced significant increase of T-regs count (CD25/CD4/Foxp3+) compared to control (5.5 vs. 2.7%, p = 0.049).

At the next step of the study we evaluated number of TLR-expressing granulocytes in PBMC cultures incubated with influenza vaccines.

All types of vaccines had immunostimulating effect on TLR-expressing cells by increasing the number of granulocytes expressing TLR 2,3,4,6,8, and 9, as shown in **Table 2**.

We found significant differences (F = 270.16, p < 0.001, q < 0.001) in the percent of granulocytes expressing TLR2 (**Table 2**, **Figure 3**) after incubation of PBMC with different types of vaccines, regardless of the AB level against the hemagglutinin of the influenza virus A/H1N1, A/H3N2 and B.. Subunit vaccine increased number of TLR2+ cells in PBMC culture from 16.6 (in control) to 38.2% (p < 0.001), adjuvanted vaccine—to 39.8% (p < 0.001), and split vaccine—to 37.5% (p < 0.001). However, there were no significant differences in TLR2 cell number between vaccine types.

Incubation of cell culture in the presence of influenza vaccines induced an increase in the number of TLR2+ granulocytes regardless of the baseline anti-influenza AB level (F = 53.25, p < 0.001, q < 0.001 – low AB level, F = 169.63, p < 0.001, q < 0.001 – medium AB level, F = 103.89, p < 0.001, q < 0.001 – high AB level) (**Figure 4**). In women with low AB level, the number

TLR	N	TLR-expressing granulocytes, %, Me (Q1-Q3)				F	p	q
		Control	Subunit	Adjuvanted	Split			
2	24	16.6 (14.2–18.38)	38.2 (36.45–40.05)	39.35 (37.73–42.4)	37.5 (35.38–39.27)	270.16	<0.001	<0.001
4	24	22.3 (19.75–25.4)	26.85 (25.23–29.43)	24.45 (22.15–26.9)	23.35 (21.5–25.35)	10.62	<0.001	<0.001
3	24	20.2 (18.23–22.95)	20 (18.02–24.05)	21.7 (19.5–23.05)	24.15 (21.95–25.95)	6.90	<0.001	<0.001
9	24	11.95 (9.825–12.85)	19.85 (17.95–25.2)	25.45 (24–26.32)	26.4 (24.48–28.23)	86.57	<0.001	<0.001
8	24	20.6 (18.68–22.4)	32.7 (30.12–35)	42.5 (37–45.1)	34.4 (29–37)	138.59	<0.001	<0.001
6	23	4.3 (4.05–5.15)	6.5 (5.95–7)	5.7 (5.2–6.9)	6.9 (5.95–7.55)	18.04	<0.001	<0.001

Table 2. Number of TLR-expressing granulocytes after incubation with influenza vaccines.

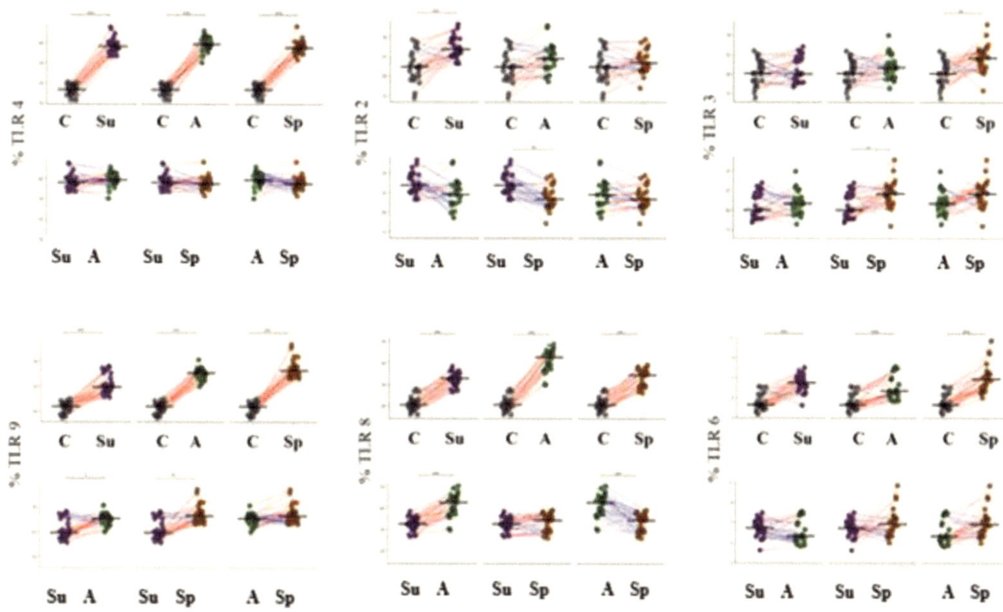

Figure 3. Number of TLR-expressing granulocytes in PBMC cultures incubated with influenza vaccines. C = control; Su = inactivated subunit influenza vaccine; A = trivalent inactivated polymer-subunit influenza vaccine; Sp = inactivated split-product influenza vaccine.

of TLR2-expressing granulocytes increased 2.4-fold after incubation with subunit vaccine ($p_h = 0.019$), 2.3-fold after incubation with adjuvanted vaccine ($p_h = 0.019$), and 2.2-fold after incubation with split vaccine ($p_h = 0.003$) compared with control.

In women with medium AB level, there was similar increase in the number of these cells: 2.3-fold for subunit and split vaccines ($p_h < 0.001$), and 2.4-fold for adjuvanted vaccine ($p_h = 0.001$) compared with control.

In women with high AB level, the number of TLR2-expressing granulocytes increased 2.6-fold after incubation with subunit vaccine ($p_h = 0.031$), 2.8-fold after incubation with adjuvanted vaccine ($p_h = 0.029$), and 2.7-fold after incubation with split vaccine ($p_h = 0.029$) compared with control.

Analysis revealed significant differences ($F = 10.62$, $p < 0.001$, $q < 0.001$) in the percent of granulocytes expressing TLR4 after incubation of PBMC with different types of vaccines, regardless of the AB level against the hemagglutinin of the influenza virus (**Table 2**, **Figure 3**). Subunit vaccine increased number of TLR4+ cells 1.2-fold compared to control ($p < 0.001$) and 1.1-fold compared to split vaccine ($p < 0.001$).

Statistically significant changes in the number of TLR4+ cells (**Figure 4**) between vaccine types were demonstrated only in women with medium AB level ($F = 5.24$, $p = 0.008$, $q = 0.010$): the number of these cells increased 1.1-fold after incubation with subunit vaccine compared to control ($p_h = 0.047$) and 1.2-fold compared to split vaccine ($p = 0.007$).

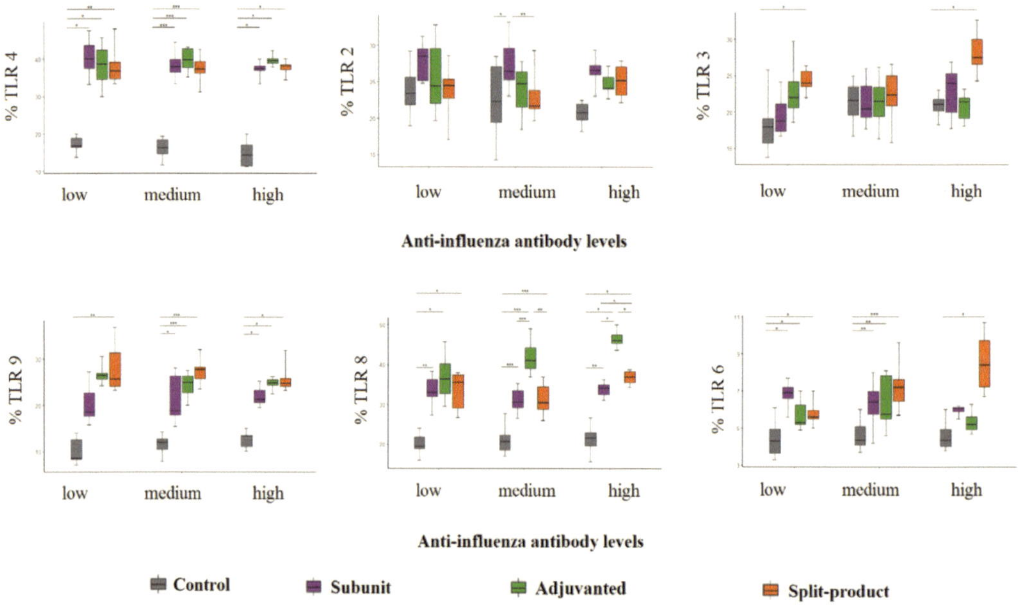

Figure 4. The impact of influenza vaccines on TLR-expressing granulocytes in PBMC cultures from volunteers with different AB titers against the hemagglutinin of the influenza virus A/H1N1, A/H3N2 and B.

Analysis of TLR3-expressing granulocytes (**Table 2**, **Figure 3**) revealed significant differences ($F = 6.90$, $p < 0.001$, $q < 0.001$) between groups, meaning that activation of the innate immunity effectors was dependent of the vaccine type, but not baseline AB level. There were significant differences for split vaccines compared to control (1.2-fold increase, $p = 0.001$) and subunit vaccine (1.2-fold increase, $p = 0.008$). That means that split vaccine had higher activity.

In women with low and high AB level, there were significant changes in the number of TLR3-expressing cells (**Figure 4**). The significance of differences was ($F = 6.05$, $p = 0.025$, $q = 0.030$) for low AB level and ($F = 6.45$, $p = 0.008$, $q = 0.010$) for high AB level. In women with low and high AB level, percent of TLR3-expressing granulocytes significantly increased after incubation with split vaccine (1.3-fold, $p_h = 0.042$ and $p_h = 0.050$, respectively) compared to control.

Analysis also revealed (**Table 2**, **Figure 3**) that different vaccines influenced ($F = 86.57$, $p < 0.001$, $q < 0.001$) the number of TLR9-positive cells regardless of the AB level. All types of vaccines increased the number of TLR9-expressing granulocytes in PBMC culture. Subunit vaccine caused 1.6-fold increase ($p < 0.001$), adjuvanted vaccine caused 2.1-fold increase ($p < 0.001$), and split vaccine caused 2.2-fold increase ($p < 0.001$) compared to control. Subunit vaccine was 1.2-fold less effective than adjuvanted vaccine ($p = 0.012$) and 1.3-fold less effective than split vaccine ($p = 0.003$).

Analysis showed that effect of different types of vaccines on TLR9-positive cells depended on the baseline AB level ($F = 26.93$, $p < 0.001$, $q < 0.001$ – low AB level; $F = 39.81$, $p < 0.001$, $q < 0.001$ – medium AB level; $F = 29.41$, $p < 0.001$, $q < 0.001$ – high AB level) (**Figure 4**). In women with low AB level, split vaccine induced threefold increase in the number of TLR9+ granulocytes compared to PBMC culture without stimulation ($p_h = 0.002$). However, in women with medium and high AB level, other types of vaccines stimulated TLR9+ granulocytes. There were following differences between vaccine types: subunit vaccine caused 1.6-fold increase ($p_h = 0.017$, $p_h = 0.050$), adjuvanted vaccine caused 2- and 1.8-fold increase ($p_h < 0.001$, $p_h = 0.040$), and split vaccine caused 2.3- and 1.8-fold increase ($p_h < 0.001$, $p_h = 0.050$) compared to control, respectively, in women with medium and high AB level.

Analysis of TLR8-expressing cells showed interesting results (**Table 2**, **Figure 3**). This receptor plays important role in recognition of viral single-stranded RNA. Analysis revealed a significant increase in the number of these cells in PBMC culture dependent on vaccine type ($F = 138.59$, $p < 0.001$, $q < 0.001$). All vaccines induced increase in the number of TLR8-positive granulocytes. This parameter increased 1.6-fold after incubation with subunit vaccine ($p < 0.001$), twofold after incubation with adjuvanted vaccine ($p < 0.001$), and 1.7-fold after incubation with split vaccine ($p < 0.001$) compared to control. Adjuvanted vaccine was 1.3-fold more effective than subunit vaccine ($p < 0.001$) and 1.2-fold more effective than split vaccine ($p < 0.001$).

Differences in the number of TLR8+ cells dependent on vaccine type were detected in all groups of volunteers, regardless of the baseline anti-influenza AB level ($F = 35.99$, $p < 0.001$, $q < 0.001$ – low AB level, $F = 76.10$, $p < 0.001$, $q < 0.001$ – medium AB level, $F = 116.13$, $p < 0.001$, $q < 0.001$ – high AB level) (**Figure 4**). In women with low, medium and high serum AB level, subunit vaccine induced 1.7-fold ($p_h < 0.001$), 1.5-fold ($p_h < 0.001$), and 1.6-fold ($p_h = 0.002$) increase, respectively, adjuvanted vaccine caused 1.9-fold ($p_h < 0.014$), twofold ($p_h < 0.001$), and 2.1-fold ($p_h = 0.014$) increase, respectively, and split vaccine caused 1.8-fold ($p_h < 0.029$), 1.5-fold ($p_h < 0.001$), and 1.7-fold ($p_h = 0.042$) increase of TLR8-expressing granulocyte number, respectively, compared to control. In women with medium and high serum AB level, immunoadjuvant-containing vaccine was, respectively, 1.3- and 1.2-fold more effective than split vaccine ($p_h = 0.002$ and $p_h = 0.042$), and 1.3-fold more effective than subunit vaccine ($p_h < 0.001$ и $p_h = 0.042$). In women with medium and high serum AB level, immunoadjuvant-containing vaccine was, respectively, 1.3- and 1.2-fold more effective than split vaccine ($p_h = 0.002$ and $p_h = 0.042$), and 1.3-fold more effective than subunit vaccine ($p_h < 0.001$ и $p_h = 0.042$).

Changes in the distribution of TLR6-expressing granulocytes were similar (**Table 2**, **Figure 3**). Analysis showed significant increase in the number of these cells in PBMC cultures dependent on vaccine type ($F = 18.04$, $p < 0.001$, $q < 0.001$). TLR6-expressing granulocyte number increased 1.5-fold after incubation with subunit vaccine, 1.3-fold after incubation with adjuvanted vaccine, and 1.6-fold after incubation with split vaccine compared to control ($p < 0.001$). However, there were no statistically significant differences between various types of vaccines.

Analysis also showed that effect of different types of vaccines on TLR6-positive cells depended on the baseline AB level ($F = 26.38$, $p < 0.001$, $q < 0.001$ – low AB level; $F = 11.71$, $p < 0.001$, $q < 0.001$ – medium AB level; $F = 16.57$, $p = 0.001$, $q = 0.001$ – high AB level) (**Figure 4**). In women with low and medium serum AB level, subunit vaccine induced 1.6-fold ($p_h = 0.043$) and 1.5-fold ($p_h = 0.004$) increase, respectively, adjuvanted vaccine caused 1.2-fold ($p_h = 0.032$) and 1.3-fold ($p_h = 0.004$) increase, respectively, and split vaccine caused 1.3-fold ($p_h = 0.027$) and 1.6-fold ($p_h < 0.001$) increase of TLR6-expressing granulocyte number, respectively, compared to control.

In women with high serum AB level, the number of TLR6-expressing granulocytes increased only after incubation with split vaccine ($p_h = 0.050$).

4. Discussion

Considering that inactivated influenza vaccines have a number of drawbacks (lack of efficacy in certain patients [1–7], no protection against drift influenza viruses [8–11]), there is a need for next generation vaccines to be developed. Besides, the effect many influenza vaccines have on the cellular and molecular immunologic mechanisms remains poorly studied.

The effects of inactivated influenza vaccines on key effectors of innate and acquired immunity are being investigated at the Mechnikov Research Institute of Vaccines and Sera (Moscow). Various types of influenza vaccines were selected for the study. First, their effect on distribution pattern of lymphocyte subpopulations was estimated *in vitro*.

Analysis of the vaccine effect on the immunophenotype of lymphocytes cultured for 72 hours, showed activation of the innate and acquired immunity effectors: NK cells (CD16/56), NKT cells (CD3/CD16/56), B lymphocytes (CD45/CD20), cells with early activation marker (CD45/CD25), T lymphocytes with late activation marker (CD3/HLA-DR), and regulatory T cells (Tregs, CD4/CD25/Foxp3). In view of this, below are characteristics of the cells that most actively responded to influenza vaccines added to PBMC culture.

Natural killer cells are essential to the innate immunity in influenza. Their function is to lyze tumor and virus-infected cells and to regulate innate and adaptive immune responses [19, 20]. Natural killer cells have been reported to identify influenza-infected cells through the NKp44 and NKp46 receptors that bind influenza hemagglutinin. Natural killer cells have also been reported to stimulate cellular immune response, regulate eosinophil maturation, and protect respiratory epithelium [21]. When interacting with peripheral mononuclear cells, PO, a component of the adjuvanted vaccine, significantly increases NK cells' cytotoxic effect on target cells. The phenomenon was observed almost in all donors examined, with the increased effect being especially pronounced in patients with the baseline activity of NK cells at the lower normal limit or decreased [22].

Being phenotypically heterogenous, NKT cells duplicate the functions of NK cells and link innate and acquired immunity [23].

Cytotoxic T lymphocytes identify and kill virus-infected cells. Infected cells present virus core antigens coupled to MHC class I molecules, which ensures their identification and subsequent killing by cytotoxic T lymphocytes [24, 25].

Specific cytotoxic lymphocytes cannot prevent cells from being initially infected with the virus, but they can restrict virus reproduction and enhance virus elimination out of the body. In unvaccinated adults, cytotoxic lymphocytes are crucial for clearing the body from influenza. They release perforin and stimulate apoptosis of virus-infected cells [26, 27].

Efficacy of influenza vaccines is currently assessed from their ability to activate the humoral immune response, as recommended in WHO guidelines. We think that this assessment does not adequately reflect the mechanisms of immune response to viruses. Therefore, it is essential to also study the cellular immunity. Immunodominance, which means that the immune system chooses one or more key epitopes for recognition, is an important factor for the development of vaccines stimulating the cellular immune response [28]. Vaccines aimed at producing cytotoxic T lymphocytes specific for an immunodominant epitope can significantly narrow the cross-reactive range of immune response to various virus strains. The role of antigen delivery route and presentation should also be considered when developing such vaccines. To stimulate a strong cytotoxic immune response, an antigen should be processed and presented by dendritic cells and coupled to MHC class I molecules. These may occur either at the moment dendritic cells are being infected or transduced or when dendritic cells engulf apoptotic bodies from other infected cells. Thus, the induction of cytotoxic immune response varies from strong one (with live attenuated vaccines) to a weaker, lower one (with inactivated whole-virion and subunit vaccines) [21].

B lymphocytes are among the key adaptive immunity effectors in influenza, since they produce anti-hemagglutinin (HA) (mainly against its globular domain) virus-neutralizing antibodies that prevent hemagglutinin from interacting with cellular receptors. Moreover, their Fc portion contributes to virion phagocytosis and to stimulation of antibody-dependent cellular cytotoxicity. HA amino acid sequence homology is about 80% between different strains within one subtype and 40–70% between strains of different subtypes. Besides, anti-neuraminidase antibodies have protective properties. They do not offer virus-neutralizing activity but they can inhibit neuraminidase enzymatic activity, which prevents the virus from spreading. Anti-neuraminidase antibodies also stimulate antibody-dependent cellular cytotoxicity. In addition, anti-neuraminidase antibodies have been shown to protect mice from H5N1 influenza virus [29].

Our study showed high stimulating effect of all studied influenza vaccines on B cell counts in PBMC culture. Adjuvanted vaccine was 1.3-fold more effective than subunit vaccine and 1.1-fold more effective than split vaccine. That means that adjuvanted vaccine activated B cell proliferation more effectively than the inactivated vaccines studied.

B cells were found to produce IgA, IgG, and IgM antibody isotypes in primary infection, while no production of IgM antibodies was observed in secondary infection. IgM antibodies are capable of activating the complement cascade as well as of neutralizing the virus [21, 29]. Secretory immunoglobulins A protect respiratory mucosae, through which influenza enters the body, and are indicative of recent virus exposure. Immunoglobulins G ensure the longest protection against influenza [21, 30].

Comparative analysis of the vaccines studied showed that adjuvanted vaccine is more effective in stimulating NK, NKT cells and Tregs, as well. The vaccine was 1.3- and 1.1-fold more effective than subunit and split vaccines in increasing NK cell count, 2.1- and 1.5-fold for NKT cell count, 1.3- and 1.16-fold for B lymphocyte count, and 1.5- and 1.2-fold for Treg count, respectively. The studied vaccines were not found to activate other cell types.

Natural thymus-derived regulatory cells (nTreg) of CD4 + CD25+ surface phenotype with constitutive expression of Foxp3 transcription factor responsible for their regulatory activity are one of the best documented cell population. Increased Treg number can possibly be explained by the immunoregulatory effect of PO (adjuvant)-containing vaccine. Immunoregulatory function of nTreg is implemented both through cytokine secretion, such as TGF-β and IL-10, and through contact interaction with the effector T lymphocytes and antigen-presenting cells [31, 32].

Innate immune mechanisms are key to protection against pathogens, since they ensure prompt inflammatory reactions including detection of highly conservative structures, which are common to many microorganisms, through special receptors of broad specificity. These are signal PRRs, and TLRs are the most important of them [33–36].

Having recognized a specific pattern, PRRs initiate a series of signal cascades, which make the first line of defense against microorganisms. Besides, these signals initiate maturation of dendritic cells, which prepare the second line of immune response to the infection, known as acquired immunity. Thus, TLRs contribute to the regulation of innate and acquired immunity. Currently known are 11 types of TLRs in humans and 13 types in mice [37, 38]. Four of them (TLR3, TLR7, TLR8, and TLR9) recognize virus RNA and DNA. TLRs have an established role in physiological regulation of pro-inflammatory cytokine production, which are required for immune response to infections caused by bacteria, fungi, and viruses [39]. Inflammation is known to be directly associated primarily with neutrophils, which express almost all identified TLRs, as it has been shown recently. This explains the importance of TLRs in neutrophil activity regulation: LPS-induced TLR4 activation induces the production of pro-inflammatory cytokines and chemokines (IL-1β, IL8, and TNFα); TLR2, TLR4, and TLR9 stimulation is accompanied by respiratory burst and changed expression of adhesion molecules [40, 41].

The study of the effect influenza vaccine has on TLR-positive cell (granulocyte) expression gave the following results.

Patients with initially different anti-influenza AT titers *in vitro* showed statistically significant differences in TLR3, TLR8, and TLR9-expressing cell counts, depending on the type of influenza vaccine added to leukocyte culture.

All the influenza vaccines studied, caused a statistically significant ($p < 0.05$) increase in TLR2-, TLR6-, TLR8-, and TLR9-positive granulocyte counts in PBMC culture, compared to non-stimulated cells.

Subunit vaccine showed statistically significant ($p < 0.001$) stimulating effect on the expression of TLR4-positive granulocytes, compared to control group and split vaccine. TLR4 is known to be an important regulator of neutrophil survival [40–42].

Split vaccine provided better increase in TLR3- ($p = 0.008$) and TLR9- ($p = 0.001$) positive cell counts, compared to subunit vaccine. Both vaccines had similar effect on TLR8+ granulocyte proliferation. TLR3 is an important receptor in recognition of viral double-stranded RNA generated during replication [43]. TLR3 expression by CD4+ и CD8+ lymphocytes is known to be accompanied by their activation, which allows them to get directly involved in various types of immune response [44].

Dendritic cell activation has been reported to occur predominantly with TLR2, TLR3, TLR4, TLR7, and TLR9. TLRs are effective contributors to APC activation, not only because they induce pro-inflammatory cytokine production, but also because they enhance expression of various co-stimulating molecules required for effective antibody recognition [45, 46]. Moreover, TLRs control dendritic cell maturation and antigen-presenting function [47].

Influenza vaccines have been reported to activate innate effectors—the first line of defense to infection—dendritic cells, both myeloid and lymphoid lineages [48]. TLR3 plays an important part in cross-priming of naive CD8 T cells that differentiate to cytotoxic T cells [49, 50]. They are key to killing virus-infected cells. TLR3 expressed on dendritic cells is also essential for NK cell activation via INAM molecule [51].

Adjuvanted vaccine showed high induction potential with respect to TLR9- and TLR8-expressing cells, compared to subunit vaccine ($p = 0.012$ and $p < 0.001$, respectively) and split vaccine ($p = 0.003$ and $p < 0.001$, respectively). TLR8 has been found to recognize viral single-stranded RNA and to be a specific receptor responsible for influenza virus recognition [45, 52]. The increased TLR8-positive cell count in this study can be attributed to the co-stimulating effect of the adjuvant in the adjuvanted vaccine.

TLR9 along with TLR2 and TLR4 are involved in the regulation of B lymphocyte activation, proliferation, differentiation, and survival (this is considered an alternative pathway of B lymphocyte activation) [53]. TLR9 is also supposed to be a PRR key to influenza identification and binding, while recognition of influenza virions by TLR7/8 is significant for the induction of protective immune response to main antigens (hemagglutinin) [54].

Two different intracellular signaling systems are generally recognized at the moment. One of them involves TLR2, TLR4, TLR5, TLR7, TLR9 and intracellular molecules MyD88, IRAK, TRAF, NFkB. This intracellular signaling system usually activates an early pro-inflammatory response. The other intracellular system involves TLR3, TLR4, (might involve TLR7 and TLR8), adaptor protein TRIF and intracellular proteins TRAM, TBK1, and IRF3. This signaling system ensures the activation of anti-virus response. TLR3 is the key component of this signaling pathway, since it interacts with double-stranded viral RNA. TLR4 is equally effective in the activation of both intracellular signaling systems. Thus, there are two important types of innate immune responses. The first type activates antibacterial protection along with the tissue inflammation. The second type provides type I interferon-mediated antiviral response, with interferon being the primary antiviral mediator in innate immunity [55].

5. Conclusion

Thus, the studies have shown that influenza vaccines activate cellular immunity effectors as well as induce humoral immune response. PO-containing adjuvanted vaccine showed the strongest capability of inducing the cellular response, among the three vaccines studied.

Influenza vaccines *in vitro* induced an increase in the number of the innate and acquired immunity effectors: NK cells, NKT cells, B lymphocytes, cells with early activation marker, T lymphocytes with late activation marker, and regulatory T cells.

Despite the fact that influenza vaccines must activate endosomal receptors, they cause nonspecific activation of the surface TLRs. This might be due to the influence exerted by antigen complexes contained in influenza vaccines of various types and due to the presence of an adjuvant in one of the vaccines studied. These vaccines activate TLR signaling cascade and, thus, can probably stimulate key effectors of the innate (DC, NK, and NKT cells) and adaptive

(CTL, B lymphocytes) immunity, which provide antiviral effect and induce body's own defense mechanisms against microbial infection.

6. Vaccination against influenza: the prospect of using adjuvants

The flu is widespread around the world and causes seasonal epidemics, which result in the death of hundreds of thousands of people each year [56]. Complications leading to morbidity and mortality following infection are predominantly observed in high-risk groups: children of early age, people with chronic diseases and pregnant women [57]. According to WHO, globally annual epidemics result in 3,000,000–5,000,000 cases of severe disease and approximately 250,000–500,000 deaths [58].

The vaccination is the most effective tools for preventing of influenza and, as a consequence, reducing the number and severity of post-infectious complications. Inactivated influenza vaccines received the most widely used, due to its high efficiency and low reactogenicity. But, at the same time, inactivated influenza vaccines, including seasonal trivalent vaccines, used for the annual prevention of influenza in the autumn-winter period, are not without some limitations. These vaccines are not enough (effective) immunogenic in vaccinating a number of population groups - small children, pregnant women, the elderly, people with various chronic diseases that are considered to be influenza risk groups. Also, inactivated influenza vaccines are not sufficiently protected against antigenically different strains (drift and heterologous) of the influenza virus that are not contained in the vaccine. In addition, the capacity of all manufacturers may not be sufficient to provide mass vaccine prevention around the world, especially in the event of a pandemic [59–61].

To increase the immunogenicity of inactivated influenza vaccines, adjuvants (immunoadjuvants) have been proposed. With the use of adjuvants, it is possible to increase the immunogenicity of influenza vaccines against a set of antigenically different strains. Adjuvants in the influenza vaccine can also provide efficacy in the immunization of various population groups, including at-risk groups. In addition, a significant increase in the immunogenicity of the vaccine due to the adjuvant will allow the transition to simple (single) immunization regimens, as well as reduce the dose of the antigen (hemagglutinin). This is especially important for pre-pandemic vaccines, because with the same production capacity, more vaccines will be obtained - and as a result, more people are immunized [59, 61].

The action of most adjuvants is based on the prolongation of the AG action, which is provided by the creation of a "depot" of the AG, which slows its absorption. Due to the sorption of AG on certain carriers, the antigen is held in places necessary for exposure of the antigen to antigen presenting cells and lymphocytes. Such an effect occurs when using aluminum alum, immunostimulating complexes, an oil microemulsion [62].

The effect of deposition is also achieved through the use of liposomes [63]. Adjuvants that primarily affect the phagocytic link of the immune system include polyelectrolytes, including PO. Structural association of the AG and polymer-immunostimulant enhances the migration of phagocytes, the functional activity of macrophages in tissues and increases their processing activity [64].

The action of adjuvants depends on the initial immune status of the organism preceding the vaccination. Adjuvants accelerate development and increase the level of immune response, increase the duration of its retention. Long rise and a slow decrease in the intensity of post-vaccination immunity is characteristic of adjuvanted vaccines. At the same time, a reliable immune response is achieved with the help of small doses of AG and a small number of injections of the vaccine [63].

PO possesses expressed immune modulating effects acting first of all on the innate immunity factors such as monocytic-macrophagal system cells, neutrophils and NK-cells and inducing their activation under initially reduced functions. Flow cytochemistry data showed that PO does interact with three lymphocyte subclasses, predominantly binds with monocytes and neutrophils and to a lesser extent with lymphocytes, enhancing intracellular H2O2 production. Hydrogen peroxide being the secondary messenger activates the transcriptional NF-kB factor that is the participant of the cytokines synthesis regulation. The enhancement of the pro-inflammatory cytokines IL-1β, IL6, TNF-α synthesis takes place. Activation by PO cells of monocytic-macrophagal cluster and natural killers promotes mobilization of both cellular and humoral immunity. Finally, all immunity starts up for adequate response development similarly to that as it occurs in natural way [65].

Besides its own clinical application as independent drug, Polyoxidonium is used as immunoadjuvant in new generation vaccines and is a compound in subunit adjuvanted Grippol family vaccines since 1997 when first Grippol® vaccine was registered in Russian market. Due to Polyoxidonium, all Grippol family vaccines contain 3-times lower antigen content in one immunizing dose - 5 mcg per strain, in comparison to 15 mcg per strain in other subunit and split influenza vaccines. This provides Grippol family vaccines with higher safety profile. Today Grippol vaccines are approved and especially recommended for vaccination of cohorts that previously were considered to be not vaccinated (patients with allergic conditions, subjects with chromic somatic diseases, individuals with different immune deficiencies), and children from 6 months of age, and pregnant women. These recommendations were made based on relevant clinical trials results followed by many years practical mass vaccine application experience [66, 67].

Annual vaccination with the "yearly adapted vaccine" is an effective means of prevention and control of influenza in immunocompetent individuals, even in those with a known poor antibody response. In addition to the development of protective antibodies after vaccination, the induction of cell-mediated immunity is considered to be of critical importance [68]. Recent researches concerning the response to influenza vaccination in patients with CVID and unclassified antibody deficiency have shown that while the humoral immune response was strongly impaired, a T cell response against the vaccine was detected in most patients [69].

Seasonal vaccines primarily work through the induction of neutralizing antibodies against the principal surface antigen HA. This important role of HA-specific antibodies explains why previous pandemics have emerged when new HAs have appeared in circulating human viruses. It has long been recognized that influenza virus-specific CD4(+) T cells are important in protection from infection through direct effector mechanisms or by providing help to B cells and CD8(+) T cells. However, the seasonal influenza vaccine is poor at inducing CD4(+) T cell responses and needs to be combined with an adjuvant facilitating this response [70].

Protective immunity induced by SF-10 (synthetic human pulmonary surfactant with a carboxy vinyl polymer as a viscosity improver) against lethal influenza virus infection was partially and predominantly suppressed after depletion of CD8+ and CD4+ T cells (induced by intraperitoneal injection of the corresponding antibodies), respectively, suggesting that CD4+ T cells predominantly and CD8+ T cells partially contribute to the protective immunity in the advanced stage of influenza virus infection [71]. These results suggest that adjuvants can promote effective antigen delivery to antigen presenting cells, activates CD8+ T cells via cross-presentation, and induces cell-mediated immune responses against antigen.

Influenza infection elicits high-affinity IgA in the respiratory tract and virus-specific IgG, which correlates with protection. Long-lived influenza-specific T cells have also been shown to ameliorate disease [72]. Activation of the parameters of innate immunity is critical for the recognition of infection, as well as for the effectiveness of vaccination, which allows not only eliminating pathogens and cells with altered antigenic properties, but also having a significant effect on the formation of adaptive immunity [73].

Development of a universal influenza vaccine currently seems to be quite workable and promising task. Such universal vaccines are expected to contain both antibody production stimulants and inductors of cellular immune response with effectors of innate and adaptive immunity being involved. Adjuvants may play an important part, their functions being aimed both at enhancing immune response to an antigen and at regulating that response [74]. Thus, due to the emergence of a new type of vaccine (adjuvant), in assessing the immunological efficacy is important not only humoral but also cellular immune response.

Conflict of interest

The authors declare no conflict of interest.

Abbreviations

CD	cluster of differentiation
PO	polyoxidonium
TLR's	toll-like receptors
WBCs	leukocytes (white blood cells)
FBS	fetal bovine serum
HAI	hemagglutination inhibition
HAU	hemagglutination unit
RBCs	red blood cells

V	Vaccine
PBMC	peripheral blood mononuclear cell
AB	Antibody
RNA	Ribonucleic acid
MHC	Major histocompatibility complex
HA	hemagglutinin
nTreg	natural thymus-derived regulatory cells
Foxp3	Forkhead box p3
TGF-β	transforming growth factor beta
IL	interleukin
PRRs	pathogen-recognize receptors
LPS	lipopolysaccarides
AG	antigen
DNA	deoxyribonucleic acid
CVID	common variable immunodeficiency
APC	antigen-presenting cell

Author details

Mikhail Petrovich Kostinov[1,2]*, Nelli Kimovna Akhmatova[1], Ekaterina Alexandrovna Khromova[1], Svetlana Anatolyevna Skhodova[1], Vera Nikolaevna Stolpnikova[1], Alexander Petrovich Cherdantsev[3] and Anna Egorovna Vlasenko[4]

*Address all correspondence to: vaccinums@gmail.com

1 I. Mechnikov Research Institute of Vaccines and Sera, Moscow, Russia

2 Federal State-Funded Educational Institution of Higher Education "First Moscow State Medical University named after I.M. Sechenov" of Ministry of Healthcare of Russia, Moscow, Russia

3 Federal State-Funded Educational Institution of Higher Education "Ulyanovsk State University", Ulyanovsk, Russia

4 Novokuznetsk State Institute of Advanced Medical Education, the Branch of Federal State-Funded Educational Institution of Additional Professional Education "Russian Medical Academy of Continuous Professional Education" of the Ministry of Healthcare of Russia, Novokuznetsk, Russia

References

[1] Gross PA, Hermogenes AW, Sacks HS, Lau J, Levandowski RA. The efficacy of influenza vaccine in elderly persons. A meta-analysis and review of the literature. Annals of Internal Medicine. 1995;**123**(7):518-527

[2] Khurana S, Frasca D, Blomberg B, Golding H. AID activity in B cells strongly correlates with polyclonal antibody affinity maturation in-vivo following pandemic 2009-H1N1 vaccination in humans. PLoS Pathogens. 2012 Sep;**8**(9):e1002920. DOI: 10.1371/journal.ppat.1002920

[3] Kositanont U, Assantachai P, Wasi C, Puthavathana P, Praditsuwan R. Kinetics of the antibody response to seasonal influenza vaccination among the elderly. Viral Immunology. 2012 Dec;**25**(6):471-476

[4] Nath KD, Burel JG, Shankar V, Pritchard AL, Towers M, Looke D, Davies JM, Upham JW. Clinical factors associated with the humoral immune response to influenza vaccination in chronic obstructive pulmonary disease. International Journal of Chronic Obstructive Pulmonary Disease. 2014;**9**:51-56

[5] Yerkovich ST, Hales BJ, Carroll ML, Burel JG, Towers MA, Smith DJ, Thomas WR, Upham JW. Reduced rhinovirus-specific antibodies are associated with acute exacerbations of chronic obstructive pulmonary disease requiring hospitalization. BMC 2012;**12**:37

[6] Pera A, Campos C, Lopez N, et al. Immunosenescence: Implications for response to infection and vaccination in older people. Maturitas. 2015;**82**:50-55

[7] Dorrington MG, Bowdish DM. Immunosenescence and novel vaccination strategies for the elderly. Frontiers in Immunology. 2013;**4**:171

[8] Belshe RB, Newman FK, Cannon J, Duane C, Treanor J, Van Hoecke C, Howe BJ, Dubin G. Serum antibody responses after intradermal vaccination against influenza. The New England Journal of Medicine 2004 Nov 25;**351**(22):2286-2294. Epub 2004 Nov 3

[9] Cox F, Roos A, Hafkemeijer N, Baart M, Tolboom J, Dekking L, Stittelaar K, Goudsmit J, Radošević K, Saeland E. Matrix-M adjuvated seasonal virosomal influenza vaccine induces partial protection in mice and ferrets against avian H5 and H7 challenge. PLoS One. 2015 Sep 24;**10**(9):e0135723. DOI: 10.1371/journal.pone.0135723

[10] Smith DJ, Lapedes AS, De Jong JC, Bestebroer TM, Rimmelzwaan GF, Osterhaus AD, Fouchier RA. Mapping the antigenic and genetic evolution of influenza virus. Science. 2004;**305**(5682):371-376. DOI: 10.1126/science.1097211

[11] Krammer F, Palese P. Advances in the development of influenza virus vaccines. Nature Reviews Drug Discovery. 2015;**14**(3):167-182

[12] Altenburg AF, Rimmelzwaan GF, de Vries RD. Virus-specific T cells as correlate of (cross-) protective immunity against influenza. Vaccine. 2015 Jan 15;**33**(4):500-506. DOI: 10.1016/j.vaccine.2014.11.054

[13] Kostinov MP, Zverev VV, editors. Vaccination against Hepatitis B, Influenza and Rubella for Adult Patients with Chronic Diseases. Practice guidelines. Moscow;2009 (in Russian)

[14] Kostinov MP, Solovyova IL. Immunomodulators and Vaccination. Moscow;2013 (in Russian)

[15] Kostinov MP. Immunocorrection of Vaccination in Persons Having Health Problems. Moscow; 2006 (in Russian)

[16] http://www.ema.europa.eu/docs/en_GB/document_library/Scientific_guideline/2009/09/WC500003945.pdf

[17] Mair P, Wilcox R. Robust Statistical Methods in R: Using the WRS2 Package. Technical report, Harvard University; 2016

[18] John H. McDonald. Handbook of Biological Statistics, 2nd edn. Baltimore, Maryland: Sparky House Publishing; 2009

[19] Yokoyama WM. Natural killer cells. In: Paul W, editor. Fundamental Immunology. Philadelphia: Lippincott, Williams & Wilkins; 2013. pp. 395-430

[20] French AR, Yokoyama WM. Natural killer cells and viral infections. Current Opinion in Immunology. 2003;**15**:45-51

[21] Paget C, Ivanov S, Fontaine J, Blanc F, Pichavant M, Renneson J, Bialecki E, Pothlichet J, Vendeville C, Barba-Speath G, Huerre MR, Faveeuw C, Si-Tahar M, Trottein F. Potential role of invariant NKT cells in the control of pulmonary inflammation and CD8+ T cell response during acute influenza A virus H3N2 pneumonia. Journal of Immunology. 2011;**186**(10):5590-5602. DOI: 10.4049/jimmunol.1002348

[22] Ivanova AS, Puchkova NG, Nekrasov AV, Gurkovskaya YaI, Apryatina VA, et al. Mechanisms of adjuvant effects of polyoxidonium. Hematopoiesis Immunology. 2015;**13**(2): 30-92 (in Russian)

[23] Constantinides MG, Bendelac A. Transcriptional regulation of the NKT cell lineage. Current Opinion in Immunology. 2013;**25**:161-167

[24] Slauenwhite D, Johnston B. Regulation of NKT cell localization in homeostasis and infection. Frontiers in Immunology. 2015;**6**:255

[25] Tupin E, Kinjo Y, Kronenberg M. The unique role of natural killer T cells in the response to microorganisms.Nat Rev. Microbiologica. 2007 Jun;**5**(6):405-417

[26] McMichael AJ, Gotch FM, Noble GR, Beare PA. Cytotoxic T-cell immunity to influenza. The New England Journal of Medicine. 1983;**309**(1):13-17. DOI: 10.1056/NEJM 198307073090103

[27] Topham DJ, Tripp RA, Doherty PC. CD8 T cells clear influenza virus by perforin or Fas-dependent processes. Journal of Immunology. 1997;**159**(11):5197-5200

[28] Yewdell JW, Bennink JR. Immunodominance in major histocompatibility complex class I-restricted T lymphocyte responses. Annual Review of Immunology. 1999;**17**:51-88

[29] Sandbulte MR, Jimenez GS, Boon AC, Smith LR, Treanor JJ, Webby RJ. Cross-reactive neuraminidase antibodies afford partial protection against H5N1 in mice and are present in unexposed humans. PLoS Medicine. 2007;**4**(2):e59. DOI: 10.1371/journal.pmed.0040059

[30] Jayasekera JP, Moseman EA, Carroll MC. Natural antibody and complement mediate neutralization of influenza virus in the absence of prior immunity. Journal of Virology. 2007;**81**(7):3487-3494. DOI: 10.1128/JVI.02128-06

[31] Kazimirko NK, Akimova EE, Zavatskiy VYu, Polyakov AS, Tatarenko DP. Immunology of normal pregnancy. Molodoy Ucheny. 2014;**3**(06):132-137 (in Russian)

[32] Kostinov MP, Khromova EA, Savis'ko AA, Kostinova AM. Functional characteristics of the immune system in normal pregnancy and their correlation with vaccination. Consilium Medicum. 2016;**18**(6):59-62 (in Russian)

[33] Willcocks S, Offord V, Seyfert HM, Coffey TJ, Werling D. Species-specific PAMP recognition by TLR2 and evidence for species-restricted interaction with Dectin-1. Journal of Leukocyte Biology. 2013 Sep;**94**(3):449-458. DOI: 10.1189/jlb.0812390

[34] Rakoff-Nahoum S, Medzhitov R. Toll-like receptors and cancer. Nature Reviews Cancer. 2009 Jan; **9**(1):57-63. DOI: 10.1038/nrc2541

[35] Kawai T, Akira S. Toll-like receptors and their crosstalk with other innate receptors in infection and immunity. Immunity. 2011;**34**:637-650

[36] Mahita J, Sowdhamini R. Investigating the effect of key mutations on the conformational dynamics of Toll-like receptor dimers through moleculardynamics simulations and protein structure networks. Proteins. 2018 Jan: 31. DOI: 10.1002/prot.25467

[37] Barreiro LB, Ben-Ali M, Quach H, Laval G, Patin E, Pickrell JK, Bouchier C, Tichit M, Neyrolles O, Gicquel B, Kidd jR, Kidd KK, Alcaïs A, Ragimbeau J, Pellegrini S, Abel L, Casa-nova JL, Quintana-Murci L. Evolutionary dynamics of human Toll-like receptors and their different contributions to host de-fense. PLoS Genetics. 2009;**5**(7):e1000562

[38] Wei T, Gong J, Rössle SC, Jamitzky F, Heckl WM, Stark RW. A leucine-rich repeat assembly approach for homology modeling of the human TLR5-10 and mouse TLR11-13 ectodomains. Journal of Molecular Modeling. 2011;**17**(1):27-36

[39] Engel A, Holt G, Lu H. The pharmacokinetics of Toll-like receptor agonists and the impact on the immune system. Expert Review of Clinical Pharmacology Journal. 2011; **4**(2):275-289

[40] Hyang LT, Paredes CJ, Papoutsakis ET, Miller WM. Gene expression analysis illuminates the transcriptional programs un-derlying the functional activity of ex vivo-expanded granulo-cytes. Physiological Genomics. 2007;**31**(1):114-125

[41] Yoshimura A, Ohishi HM, Aki D, Hanada T. Regulation of TLR signaling and inflammation by SOCS family proteins. Journal of Leukocyte Biology. 2004;**5**(3):422-427

[42] Sabroe LR, Prince EC, Jones et al. Selective roles for Toll-like receptor (TLR)2 and TLR4 in the regulation of neutrophil activation and life span. The Journal of Immunology. 2003; **170**(10):5268-5275

[43] Maitra R, Augustine T, Dayan Y, Chandy C, Coffey M, Goel S. Toll like receptor 3 as an immunotherapeutic target for KRAS mutated colorectal cancer. Oncotarget. 2017 May 23;**8**(21):35138-35135,153. DOI: 10.18632/oncotarget.16812

[44] Asprodites N, Zheng L, Geng D, Velasco-Gonzalez C, Sanchez-Perez L, Davila E. Engagement of Toll-like receptor-2 on cytotoxic T-lymphocytes occurs *in vivo* and augments antitumor activity. FASEB Journal. 2008;**22**(10):3628-3637

[45] Kawai T, Akira S. The role of pattern-recognition receptors in innate immunity: Update on Toll-like receptors. Nature Immunology. 2010 May;**11**(5):373-384

[46] Kumagai Y, Takeuchi O, Kato H, et al. Alveolar macrophages are the primary interferon-alpha producer in pulmonary infection with RNA viruses. Immunity. 2007;**27**:240-252

[47] Manicassamy S, Pulendran B. Modulation of adaptive immunity with Toll-like receptors. Seminars in Immunology. 2009 Aug;**21**(4):185-193

[48] Khromova EA, Akhmatova EA, Skhodova SA, Semochkin IA, Khomenkov VG, Akhmatova NK, Kostinov MP. Effect of influenza vaccines on subpopulations of blood dendritic cells. Journal of Microbiology, Epidemiology and Immunobiology. 2016;(5):23-28 (in Russian)

[49] Schulz O, Diebold SS, Chen M, et al. Toll-like receptor 3 promotes cross-priming to virus-infected cells. Nature. 2005;**433**:887-892

[50] Azuma M, Ebihara T, Oshiumi H, Matsumoto M, Seya T. Cross-priming for antitumor CTL induced by soluble Ag + polyI:C depends on the TICAM-1 pathway in mouse CD11c(+)/CD8α (+) dendritic cells. Oncoimmunology. 2012;**1**:581-592. DOI: 10.4161/onci.19893

[51] Kasamatsu J, Azuma M, Oshiumi H, et al. INAM plays acritical role in IFN-gamma production by NK cells interacting with polyinosinic-polycytidylic acid-stimulated accessory cells. Journal of Immunology. 2014;**193**:5199-5207

[52] Hu T, Suter SR, Mumbleau MM, Beal PA. TLR8 activation and inhibition by guanosine analogs in RNA: Importance of functional groups and chain length. Bioorganic & Medicinal Chemistry. 2018 Jan 1;**26**(1):77-83. DOI: 10.1016/j.bmc.2017.11.020

[53] Jain S, Chodisetti S, Agrewala J. CD40 signaling synergizes with TLR-2 in the BCR independent activation of resting B cells. PLoS One. 2011;**6**(6):e20651

[54] Heer A, Shamshiev A, Donda A, et al. TLR signaling fine-tunes anti-influenza B cell responses. Journal of Immunology. 2007;**178**:2182-2191

[55] Markushin SG. Specifics of innate immunity in viral infections. Epidemiology and Vaccinal Prevention. 2012;**1**(62):72-81 (in Russian)

[56] Kuiken T, Riteau B, Fouchier RA, Rimmelzwaan GF. Pathogenesis of influenza virus infections: the good, the bad and the ugly. Current Opinion in Virology. 2012;**2**(3):276-286. DOI: 10.1016/j.coviro.2012.02.013

[57] Siston AM, Rasmussen SA, Honein MA, et al. Pandemic 2009 influenza A (H1N1) virus illness among pregnant women in the United States. Journal of the American Medical Association. 2010;**303**:1517-1525

[58] WHO: Influenza Fact Sheet. http://www.who.int/mediacentre/factsheets/fs211/en/

[59] WHO. Vaccines against influenza WHO posnion paper ~ November 2012. Weekly Epidemiological Record. 2012;**87**(47):461-476

[60] WHO. Influenza vaccines WHO position paper. Weekly Epidemiological Record. 2005; **80**(33):279-287

[61] Wright P, Neumann G, Kawaoka Y. Orthomyxoviruses. In: Knipe D, Howley P, editors. Fields Virology. 6th ed. Lippincott Williams & Wilkins; 2013

[62] Nikitina TN, Avdeyeva ZhI, Alpatova NA. Study of immune adjyuvant effect of cytokines in experimental models. Cytokines and Inflammation. 2010;**9**(3):19-24 (in Russian)

[63] Medunitsyn NV. Vaccinology M: "Triada-X". 2004. 446 c. (in Russian)

[64] Petrov RV, Khaitov RM. International Journal on Immunorehabilitation. 1999;**11**:C. 13-25. (in Russian)

[65] Dyakonova VA, Dambaeva SV, Pinegin BV, Khaitov RM. Study of interaction between the polyoxidonium immunomodulator and the human immune system cells. International Immunopharmacology. 2004;**4**(13):1615-1623 (in Russian)

[66] Savelyeva GM, Sukhikh GT, Serov VN, Manukhin IB, Radzinsky VE, ediotrs. Gynecology. National Guideline. 2nd edn. Moscow: GEOTAR-Media; 2017. (in Russian)

[67] Boytsov SA, Loukianov MM, Platonova EV, Gorbunov VM, Romanchuk SW, Nazarova OA, Belova OA, Kravtsova EA, Dovgalevsky PYa, Furman NV, Mironova AA, Dolotovskaya PV, Nekrasov AV, Puchkova NG, Abramova MA, Belova EN, Klyashtorny VG, Deev AD. Efficiency of influenza vaccination in patients with circulatory system diseases under dispensary observation in outpatient clinics: prospective follow-up monitoring data. Rational Pharmacotherapy in Cardiology. 2016;**12**(6):703-710. DOI: http://dx.doi.org/10.20996/1819-6446-2016-12-6-703-710 (in Russian)

[68] Principi N, Esposito S. Vaccine use in primary immunodeficiency disorders. Vaccine. 2014;**32**:3725-3731

[69] Hanitsch LG, Lobel M, Mieves JF, Bauer S, Babel N, Schweiger B, Wittke K, Grabowski P,Volk HD, Scheibenbogen C. Cellular and humeral influenza specific immune response upon vaccination in patients with common variable immunodeficiency and unclassified antibody deficiency. Vaccine. 2016 May 5;**34**(21):2417-2423

[70] Christensen D, Christensen JP, Korsholm KS, Isling LK, Erneholm K, Thomsen AR, Andersen P. Seasonal influenza split vaccines confer partial cross-protection against

heterologous influenza virus in ferrets when combined with the CAF01 Adjuvant. Frontiers in Immunology. 2018 Jan 8;**8**:1928. DOI: 10.3389/fimmu.2017.01928 eCollection 2017

[71] Kim H, Kimoto T, Sakai S, Takahashi E, Kido H. Adjuvanting influenza hemagglutinin vaccine with a human pulmonary surfactant-mimicking synthetic compound SF-10 induces local and systemic cell-mediated immunity in mice. PLoS One. 2018 Jan 25; **13**(1):e0191133. DOI: 10.1371/journal.pone.0191133 eCollection 2018

[72] Ascough S, Paterson S, Chiu C. Induction and subversion of human protective immunity: contrasting influenza and respiratory syncytial virus. Frontiers in Immunology. 2018 Mar 2;**9**:323. DOI: 10.3389/fimmu.2018.00323 eCollection 2018

[73] Gasteiger G, D'Osualdo A, Schubert DA, Weber A, Bruscia EM, Hartl D. Cellular innate immunity: An old game with new players. Journal of Innate Immunity 2017;**9**(2):111-125. DOI: 10.1159/000453397. Epub 2016 Dec 23

[74] Esmagambetov IB, Alekseeva SV, Sayadyan Kh.S, Shmarov MM. Modern approach to creation of universal influenza vaccine. Infektsiya i Immunitet. 2016;**6**(2). DOI: http://dx.doi.org/10.15789/2220-7619-2016-2-117-132 (in Russian)

Section 6

Molecular Assessment of the Safety and Quality of Influenza Vaccines and Adjuvants

Chapter 6

Genomic Approaches Enable Evaluation of the Safety and Quality of Influenza Vaccines and Adjuvants

Eita Sasaki, Takuo Mizukami and Isao Hamaguchi

Additional information is available at the end of the chapter

http://dx.doi.org/10.5772/intechopen.76361

Abstract

Vaccination is an effective means for prevention of the progression and spread of influenza virus infection. Nonetheless, there is a risk of adverse reactions, such as pain and fever, during the vaccination. In addition, because people from a wide age range, that is, from children to the elderly, are inoculated with vaccines, safety confirmation of these vaccines is important. Safety assessments of a vaccine, in the form of quality controls, have been carried out on animals. For example, the abnormal toxicity test is based on body weight changes as a toxicity index, and the leukopenic toxicity test can evaluate hematological toxicity. Meanwhile, since the 2000s, safety evaluation of drugs and chemicals by the genomic approach has been conducted frequently. The benefits with respect to safety evaluation are high sensitivity and abundant information about toxicity profiles. In this chapter, we describe the genes that are helpful as safety assessment markers and their usefulness for safety testing and vaccine development. In addition, this information may provide toxicity profiles, help understand the reactogenicity of nasal vaccines or adjuvants, and explain the prospects of genomic analyses in the development of novel vaccines and adjuvants.

Keywords: influenza vaccine, safety test, biomarker, preclinical test, quality control

1. Introduction

The current toxicological assays for chemicals and biological therapeutics (biologicals) involve high costs, are time-consuming, and require a large number of animals. Thus, such a project becomes a substantial investment in the development of a drug or biological therapeutic [1, 2]. There is a need to improve these preexisting safety-testing strategies.

The microarray technology was recognized in the toxicology research community after its introduction in the 1990s [3–5]. Subsequently, toxicological studies using the microarray technology have given rise to a new field termed toxicogenomics [6]. By integrating the genomic technology and bioinformatics, toxicogenomics has garnered a great deal of attention as an alternative means of addressing drug safety by studying the fundamental molecular mechanism of toxicity, which was difficult to detect with conventional toxicological methods [6]. In fact, microarray-based toxicogenomics remains a major breakthrough. Using microarrays, we can monitor the expression levels of tens of thousands of genes at the same time and evaluate gene expression profiles altered by various compounds or changes in gene expression profiles associated with different physiological conditions. Moreover, testing a large number of genes together gives the opportunity to identify genetic patterns and signatures that provide unique insights into drug toxicity, which are difficult to obtain by conventional animal-based techniques [7]. Thus, toxicogenomics is expected to revolutionize the traditional approaches to toxicity assessment and has been considered a paradigm shift in toxicology. To date, many studies have revealed the value of toxicogenomics [8–15]. For example, it has been suggested that toxicogenomic biomarkers can identify drug candidates that are more likely to cause toxicity in susceptible patient populations despite the lack of conventional toxicity indicators, such as hematological parameters, body weight changes, blood biochemical data, and histopathological data, which are examined in preclinical studies [16, 17]. Similarly, more sensitive biomarkers for the detection of early toxicity can be analyzed at "subtoxic doses" of a candidate therapeutic agent, where the injury is at the genetic level, but does not occur at the phenotypic level or cannot be detected by clinical-chemistry measurements [18].

Just as chemical and synthetic drugs, biological therapeutics are evaluated for their toxicity by safety tests involving animal experiments, as part of preclinical studies. In addition, to guarantee the quality and homogeneity of the preparation, a portion of the biological preparation is subjected to toxicity tests for each lot [19, 20]. These toxicity tests are based on the aforementioned conventional assays, and phenotypic alterations such as body weight changes, hematological changes, pathological changes, and similar parameters are the evaluation criteria [19, 21]. Tests of the safety and quality control of vaccines include the abnormal toxicity test (ATT, also known as a general toxicity test) [21], and the leukopenic toxicity test (LTT) [19]. In all preclinical trials, in addition to these tests, a pathological examination is carried out. Although these tests have historically been practiced for a long time, it is expected that genomics techniques will be incorporated into these tests to improve their sensitivity and to obtain information on toxicity. For biologicals, however, toxicity studies using the genomics technology have not yet been actively carried out, when compared to the testing of chemical and synthetic drugs.

Therefore, we have been using the genomics technology to search for vaccine safety assessment markers since the late 2000s. In particular, we have been conducting research on the use of genomics technology for studying pertussis vaccine [22, 23], Japanese encephalitis vaccine [24], and influenza vaccine [25]. This chapter provides an introduction to the genomics technology in the safety assessment and quality control evaluation of influenza vaccines and describes a new evaluation method involving the biomarkers obtained by the genomics technology.

2. Current vaccine safety tests

This section describes the lot release safety and quality control testing methods implemented for the influenza vaccine. The ATT has been conventionally conducted as an animal-based test to evaluate the contamination by phenol, which is used in the process of inactivating endotoxins, viruses, and bacteria [26, 27]. The method of ATT is simple: 5 mL of a sample is injected into the abdominal cavity of a guinea pig, and its survival and 7-day body weight changes are measured [19]. It has been suggested that these 7-day body weight changes reflect the biological activity of the vaccine. Indeed, if the animals were inoculated with a different type of influenza vaccine, their body weight changes would show different profiles [21]. The whole-particle inactivated influenza vaccine (WPV) that has high reactogenicity [28]. Nevertheless, it causes highly frequent adverse reactions, such as pain, swelling, and fever [29]; on the other hand, the hemagglutinin-split influenza vaccine (HAV), whose effectiveness is inferior to that of the WPV [28], has been reported to cause almost no adverse reactions [29]. The current seasonal influenza vaccines are based on the HAV, and the WPV is manufactured only as a pandemic vaccine. This approach also includes avoiding adverse reactions caused by WPVs. Therefore, the WPV also serves as a toxicity index in the quality control testing of the HAV by the LTT, which is described later.

The LTT is a safety test that assesses the leukopenic toxicity induced by the WPV as a toxicity index [19]. In this method, mice are inoculated with 0.5 mL of a WPV as a toxicity reference vaccine, and the leukopenic activity rate induced by the WPV at that time point is set to 100% leukopenic activity. At that time point, the test sample confirms whether the leukopenic activity rate is within 20% or not. The test criterion is as follows: the leukopenic activity rate should be less than 20% of the toxicity control. On the other hand, the ATT is an assay that evaluates the body weight loss of guinea pigs, and the transition during their recovery. When the same experiment was carried out in rats, WPV-injected rats showed a severe body weight loss, unlike HAV-injected rats [21]. A vaccine showing a statistically significant body weight loss in a population, when compared with a homogeneous preparation, would be rejected in terms of its quality.

Thus, safety and quality of the HAV are mainly ensured by two tests. Safety assessments of the HAV have been conducted using WPVs, which is one of the safety indices.

3. The genomic approach to identifying novel biomarkers of influenza vaccine safety

The search for new biomarkers that can reflect the bioactivity assessed in the ATT and LTT was conducted by performing comprehensive gene expression analyses on major organs via the microarray technology [25]. Inactivated influenza vaccines have been widely used for preventing infections and the spread of infections; they can roughly be subdivided into two types: the HAV and WPV [30]. The HAV mainly contains hemagglutinin (HA). This type of vaccine has no strong bioactivity; it does not contain substances other than HA proteins that act as antigens, thereby leading to no adverse reactions. Nevertheless, their ability to induce antibody production is considered insufficient to prevent the progression of influenza virus infection [30]. Historically, however, vaccines have been more effective than the existing split vaccines. The WPV is considered effective against influenza virus infections. This type of vaccine contains the whole influenza virus particle, including lipid and single-stranded RNA, and therefore, drives various immune responses. On the other hand, various WPV-induced immune responses also cause adverse reactions in humans [29]. Therefore, although WPV is a highly effective vaccine, it has lately not been employed as a seasonal influenza vaccine and is only partially manufactured as a pandemic influenza vaccine. We have carried out the searches for safety assessment marker genes of the HAV using two types of vaccines: the WPV and split influenza vaccine (SV). The WPV has high reactogenicity (effectiveness and toxicity) and therefore serves as a toxicity reference. The SV has low reactogenicity and frequency of adverse reactions and is therefore employed as a safety control. As a result, the clearest clustering of gene expression patterns in the lungs of animals by different types of vaccines was obtained [25]. In particular, the gene expression patterns in the lungs differed between the SV-treated and WPV-treated animals. Furthermore, the gene expression levels, which showed large differences between the SV- and WPV-treated animals, were estimated. As a result, 18 genes expressed in the lungs were identified as biomarker genes (**Table 1**) [25].

Symbol	Official full name	Accession
Cxcl11	Chemokine (C-X-C motif) ligand 11	NM_019494
Cxcl9	Chemokine (C-X-C motif) ligand 9	NM_008599
Zbp1	Z-DNA binding protein 1	NM_021394
Mx2	MX dynamin-like GTPase 2	NM_013606
Irf7	Interferon regulatory factor 7	NM_016850
Lgals9	Lectin, galactoside-binding, soluble, 9	NM_010708
Ifi47	Interferon gamma inducible protein 47	NM_008330
Tapbp	TAP binding protein (tapasin)	NM_001025313
Csf1	Colony stimulating factor (macrophage)	NM_007778
Timp1	Tissue inhibitor of metalloproteinase 1	NM_001044384
Trafd1	TRAF type zinc finger domain containing 1	NM_001163470
Lgals3bp	Lectin, galactoside-binding, soluble, 3 binding protein	NM_011150
Psmb9	Proteasome (prosome and macropain) subunit, beta type, 9	NM_013585
C2	Complement component 2	NM_013484
Tap2	Transporter 2, ATP-binding cassette, sub-family B (MDR/TAP)	XM_006525355
Ifrd1	Interferon-related developmental regulator 1	NM_013562
Psme1	Proteasome (prosome and macropain) activator subunit 1	NM_011189
Ngfr	Nerve growth factor receptor	NM_033217

Table 1. Marker genes for safety evaluation of influenza vaccines.

Functionally, these biomarker genes tend to correlate with the white blood cell (WBC) count in the peripheral blood of animals (leukopenic toxicity) that were treated with the inactivated influenza vaccine [31, 32]. It has been known that intraperitoneal injection of the WPV causes leukopenic toxicity in mice, and this bioactivity has been used as an index for the safety evaluation of inactivated influenza vaccines in Japan, which is termed the LTT [19]. In addition, WPV-induced body weight loss may be reflected in biomarker gene expression levels [25]. Thus, WPV-like bioactivity assessed by the ATT could be predicted by the expression levels of biomarker genes. Furthermore, the biomarker genes can partially measure biological activities that cannot be quantitated by means of body weight changes. For example, the identified biomarker gene expression increases with leukopenia and weight loss; however, some genes show increased expression even in a state without body weight loss and without a decreased WBC count (without leukopenic toxicity) [33]. The SV hardly induces the elevated expression of biomarker genes. By contrast, if SVs produced at different manufacturing plants were evaluated using the biomarker gene expression levels, variations in their quality can be reflected in the expression levels [33]. This variation is not indicated by body weight changes or by the WBC count [33]. This case is an example where the gene expression level can detect biological reactions that cannot be detected by phenotypic changes. This is the advantage of the toxicogenomics technology. Thus, it is likely that the genomics technology is also useful for the safety assessment of vaccines. Furthermore, there is a possibility that the assay involving the newly identified biomarker genes can be widely adopted as an alternative method to the currently popular methods: the ATT and LTT.

4. Safety evaluation of influenza vaccines on the basis of biomarker gene expression

The utility of the identified biomarker genes has been verified. For seasonal influenza vaccines, the ATT has been regarded as a test for safety and quality control. Therefore, a safety assessment of SVs manufactured at four manufacturing plants was conducted by means of biomarker gene expression and body weight as parameters (ATT) and by the LTT, with a WPV as a control [33]. With respect to phenotypic changes, body weight loss rates of all the SVs were found to be equivalent, and leukocyte number reduction was hardly observed for the HAVs from all the manufacturers. Nevertheless, in case of one manufacturer's HAV, analyses of the expression of 18 biomarker genes in lungs showed a significant difference in gene expression levels from other manufacturers' HAV [33]. This result suggests that the biomarker genes identified by the microarray analysis can capture biological changes that cannot be detected by body weight changes and leukocyte number reductions. This finding indicates that the analysis of expression of biomarker genes is a more sensitive assay than the conventional safety and quality control tests (ATT and LTT). This evaluation method can be applied not only to predict the toxicity but also to evaluate the homogeneity among vaccines produced in different batches.

Subsequently, the safety assessment of trivalent virosome-type influenza vaccine (Inflexal Berna V) currently licensed in several European countries such as Switzerland and Italy was performed by means of the biomarker genes. The virosome-type influenza vaccine is similar to the WPV but does not contain viral RNA. Leukopenic reactions were not noticeable when the animals were vaccinated with the virosome-type influenza vaccine; however, a body weight loss was observed, accompanied by an increase in the expression of some biomarker genes [31]. It is thought that some biological activities of this vaccine may be close to those of the WPV, because just like the WPV, Inflexal Berna V consists of a virosomal formulation. Genes whose increased expression levels were induced by the virosomal type influenza vaccine include *Tap2* and *Psmb9*, which are involved in antigen presentation and antigen digestion, suggesting that the antigen-presenting ability is higher for the virosomal-type influenza vaccine than for the HAV [31]. Consequently, it is likely that biomarker genes obtained by genomic analysis can elucidate the mechanistic details of bioactivity and toxicity.

5. Safety evaluation of the nasal influenza vaccine using biomarker gene expression

Nasal vaccines have been attracting attention as promising strategies against influenza virus infection. This is because nasal vaccines can predominantly induce mucosal immunity, when compared with conventional subcutaneous vaccines or intramuscularly injectable vaccines [34]. In nasal vaccines, IgA antibody production and secretion in the bronchial and intranasal cavities are observed, and this approach seems to be effective for the prevention of influenza infection [35–37]. For this reason, several newly developed vaccines have been designed on the premise of nasal inoculation. It is important to develop a safety assessment method for nasal vaccines by assays that are different from the conventional intramuscular and subcutaneous injections. This is because there are case control studies on the use of the inactivated intranasal influenza vaccine, which is composed of influenza antigens in a virosomal formulation with an *E. coli*-derived LT adjuvant, and the risk of Bell's palsy in Switzerland [38]. Therefore, to determine the relation between the expression of the 18 biomarker genes and the safety evaluation of the nasal inoculation influenza vaccine, an assay was devised. Mice were nasally inoculated with an influenza vaccine, and biomarker gene expression levels in the lungs were analyzed [39]. As described earlier, this biomarker gene has been identified based on the gene expression profile obtained when the vaccine was inoculated intraperitoneally. After the administration of the nasal influenza vaccines, there was an increase in the WPV-dependent expression of the biomarker gene; the evaluation of the HAV based on WPV was shown to be possible by nasal inoculation and by analysis of marker genes [39]. Furthermore, the biomarker expression level positively correlated with lymphoproliferation in nasal-associated lymphoid tissue [39], and it was inferred that this formulation induces the activity of mucosal immunity. Furthermore, in recent years, the development of an adjuvant-containing vaccine has been advanced for the purpose of enhancing the effectiveness of SVs [37]. The same trend in nasal vaccines has also been seen [37] because of the ability to induce IgA production by SVs alone is not enough to prevent infection with an influenza virus. Therefore, there has been active development of adjuvanted influenza vaccines. Although adjuvants increase the effectiveness of vaccines, strong adjuvant bioactivity is thought to lead to toxicity.

The strong bioactivity of the adjuvant will ensure increased effectiveness of vaccines. In some cases, however, highly reactogenic adjuvants can cause toxicity in humans. For example, poly I:C is known to function as an excellent vaccine adjuvant. On the other hand, it is known to cause exothermic reactions and cytokine storms [40–42]. Additionally, in the past, poly I:C has been discontinued due to adverse reactions such as a fever and arthritis in clinical trials [40]. Even other adjuvants such as R848, a Toll-like receptor (TLR)7/8 agonist, are known to cause cold-like symptoms, including a fever [43–45]. Such compounds are **excellent in terms of enhancing the** effectiveness of the vaccine; however, the risk of developing toxicity remains high. Therefore, we hypothesized that the expression of 18 biomarker genes could be applied to the safety assessment of adjuvanted vaccines. The objective of this safety test is to identify an adjuvant that has high reactogenicity and toxicity such as poly I:C and R848. The risks of adverse reactions caused by adjuvanted vaccines as test products were compared with those of the WPV. In the case of a nasal vaccine, expression of some biomarker genes was higher when animals were inoculated with the TLR9 agonist CpG K3-adjuvanted HAV, than when the animals were inoculated with the HAV alone [39]. Nonetheless, the marker gene expression levels were markedly lower than those of the WPV. Thus, the CpG K3 adjuvant did not have high reactogenicity accompanied by toxicity. The CpG K3 adjuvant is under development for use with malaria vaccines [46]; no adverse reactions have been reported so far. The authors of these reports presumed that the risk of toxicity would not be high in humans. Currently, the authors are working on building a database for constructing an adjuvant evaluation system based on an influenza vaccine that includes various adjuvants including poly I:C and R848, an oil/water emulsion adjuvant, and various other TLR-related adjuvants.

6. Development of an alternative assay for the leukopenic toxicity test based on biomarker gene expression

The biomarker genes for the safety assessment of an influenza vaccine are characterized by the biological activity that can be detected by the ATT and LTT. Specifically, biomarker gene expression levels and the WBC count with body weight changes show a negative correlation [31]. Momose *et al.* (2015) reported that a virosomal influenza vaccine caused only a body weight loss and did not cause leukopenia; however, some of the marker genes showed increased expression levels at that time point [31]. In other words, it seems that all the marker genes cannot respond uniformly via the same mechanism of action. Therefore, we considered whether the leukocytopenic activity could be evaluated with the expression of the marker genes responsible for the leukopenic activity, and we searched for biomarker genes associated with leukocytopenic activity. Furthermore, we devised a method for WBC count-predicting systems involving only the biomarker gene expression levels. If this method is established, it will be possible to set up the WBC number prediction using the biomarker gene expression and body weight loss evaluation by the ATT in one test system. This strategy will reduce the number of animals required and shorten the testing duration. We tried to identify the genes useful for the prediction of the WBC count from the biomarker gene set by multiple linear regression analysis and a stepwise method [32]. In the multiple regression analysis method, a linear equation expressed by the following formula was derived, and a predicted value was calculated. In particular, the leukocyte count of the animals and data on the expression levels of all the biomarker genes were acquired. The animals were inoculated with the WPV or HAV, and the expression levels of marker genes and numbers of WBCs were then determined. Multiple regression analysis was performed on the acquired data. A linear equation was then derived. The regression equation is shown below.

$$\text{(Predicted WBC)} = \text{(intercept)} + \beta_1 x_1 + \beta_2 x_2 + \ldots + \beta_n x_n \quad (1)$$

In this equation, "x" is substituted by the marker gene expression that corresponds to its coefficient (β); "n" indicates the number of factors corresponding to the number of selected genes. The intercept was used for calculation of the WBC number in the multiple regression analysis.

Precision of the prediction differs depending on the combination of marker genes. Therefore, by the stepwise method, a linear equation was derived that contains the combinations of marker genes having the highest prediction accuracy. As a result, some gene combinations (models) were selected (**Table 2**). Predicted leukocyte numbers produced by these models can predict leukopenia caused by WPVs with high accuracy (**Figure 1**). Even if the predicted

Predictor variable	**Model 1**	**Model 2**	**Model 3**	**Model 4**
	β	β	β	β
Intercept	2141.2	5390.6	4222.5	5293.7
C2	—	—	—	502.8
Trafd1	−3196.2	−2886.6	—	−1131.1
Irf7	—	—	—	−94.7
Csf1	—	—	—	1118.1
Ngfr	−1344.8	—	—	−360.1
Ifi47	—	—	—	472.3
Ifrd1	—	—	—	−1628.5
Psme1	4099.9	—	—	—
Tap2	3084.6	1839.1	—	—
Cxcl11	−0.3847	−0.1217	—	—
Lgals9	−8.0607	—	—	—
Zbp1	−197.49	—	—	—
Cxcl9	—	—	1.8226	—
Lgals3bp	—	—	−552.93	—
Tapbp	—	—	349.20	—

Table 2. Multiple regression by the stepwise forward selection method for the leukopenic reaction prediction model (cells/μl blood).

values of individuals are analyzed, the deviation between the predicted value and the measured value is small [32]. In addition, variations in the WBC count owing to individual differences are reproduced with high accuracy [32]. Therefore, it was shown that the leukopenic activity can be predicted by means of the identified marker gene set. With this method, it is expected that it will be possible to carry out WBC count reduction assays and abnormal toxicity negative tests by expression analysis of one biomarker gene. As mentioned in the previous section, the development of adjuvanted vaccines has advanced in recent years. Some adjuvants, like WPVs, exert a leukocytopenic activity. Leukopenic activity is also present in compounds with an excellent adjuvant activity such as Poly I:C and R848 [43]. Therefore, we analyzed the CpG K3 adjuvant, which manifested a slight leukopenic activity according to the newly developed multiple regression Equation [32]. As a result, a slight leukopenic activity was observed in animals that received the CpG K3 adjuvant in combination with the SV. Furthermore, when the expression levels of the marker genes were analyzed, and the predicted WBC count was calculated from their expression levels, the leukocyte count reduction by the CpG K3 adjuvant could be predicted with high accuracy [32]. At the same time, however, it became clear that leukocytosis is unpredictable in this system [32]. When the CpG K3 adjuvant was inoculated at low concentrations, the leukocyte count tended to

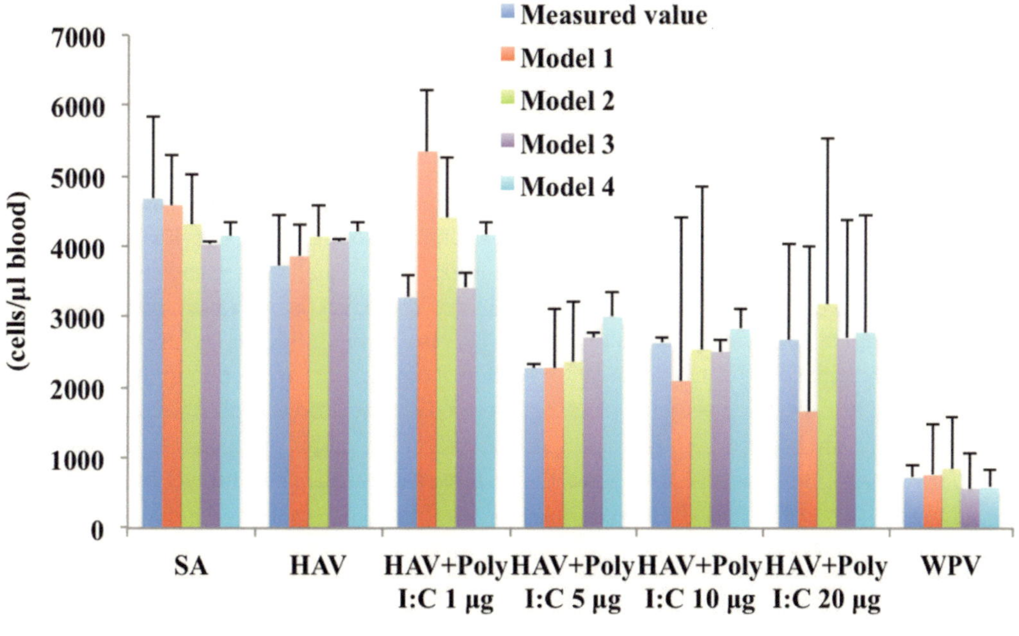

Figure 1. Prediction of a leukocyte count reduction by means of marker gene expression levels in mice treated with influenza vaccine. In the leukopenic toxicity test (LTT), mice were intraperitoneally injected with 0.5 mL of one of influenza vaccines. The dosing of whole-particle inactivated influenza vaccine (WPV) and hemagglutinin-split vaccine (HAV) was 15 µg hemagglutinin (HA)/0.5 mL. Poly I:C was reconstituted in an appropriate volume of the HAV solution to obtain concentrations of 1, 5, 10, and 20 µg poly I:C per dose. Saline (SA) served as the cssssontrol. Sixteen hours after vaccination, blood was collected to assess the numbers of leukocytes, and the lungs were immediately excised. The collected lung tissue was subjected to gene expression analyses. The predicted values were calculated via the multiple regression equation. The coefficient values and values serving as the intercept are indicated in **Table 2**. The error bar indicates standard deviation.

increase. This increase in the WBC count could not be predicted from the biomarker gene expression levels. The possible reason is that multiple linear regression analysis was performed on the animals inoculated with vaccines with leukopenic activity. The physiological association of the extracted biomarker gene with leukopenia could be another reason for this phenomenon. We have identified biomarker genes highly correlating with leukocyte counts in mathematical terms, ignoring the functions of the genes. There is a report that apoptosis of leukocytes caused by type 1 interferons (IFNs) could be a mechanism underlying the WBC count reduction by WPVs [47]. The marker gene set contains many genes related to type 1 IFN. By contrast, in model 4 (**Table 2**), more than a half of the genes related to type 1 IFN were omitted because they lacked predictability. As a result, it is conceivable that a correlation cannot be obtained from only a simple expression level because of the time lag between gene expression and actual leukocyte depletion; furthermore, a gene itself forms a complicated network.

7. Possibility of application of genomic approaches to *in vitro* safety evaluation methods

Currently, safety evaluation and parts of quality control of vaccines are carried out in animal experiments. The ATT and LTT are representative tests in this regard; they have been practiced for more than 50 years [48]. Due to the nature of the test, the ATT excludes the unintended toxicity of the vaccine; the test of lots having reactogenicity different from that of other reference lots is a final confirmatory test designed to prevent serious toxicity in humans [21]. Actually, the ATT has been incorporated into the lot release of vaccines, especially for inactivated influenza vaccines in Japan [19]. On the other hand, tests on animals are being replaced with *in vitro* evaluation systems involving cultured cells, from the viewpoint of animal welfare and cost [48]. In the safety evaluation of chemically synthesized medicines, there has been a notable development: human cultured hepatocytes and cardiomyocytes prepared from induced pluripotent stem cells [48–52]. The benefit of the *in vitro* evaluation system is not only the reduction in the number of animals used, but also the possibility of using human tissue or fluid samples, so that extrapolation to humans can be expected. For biologicals, a part of the rabbit pyrogen test was replaced with an endotoxin quantitative test. Nevertheless, this replacement has not yet been achieved for all biologicals. The endotoxin test could not be performed on some preparations because of the presence of interfering substances [53, 54]. Therefore, a rabbit pyrogen test has been carried out for these biologicals. In this test, the causative agent of the fever has been recognized as the endotoxin in some biologicals. Thus, switching to a method of directly quantitating endotoxins was introduced as an alternative for the rabbit pyrogen test. Nonetheless, because the ATT evaluates the weight loss of animals, it is difficult to determine from body weight changes what types of molecular signaling pathways or physiological reactions have been affected. Therefore, it has not been easy to develop an *in vitro* assay as an alternative for the ATT.

We have tried to create a safety evaluation system for an influenza vaccine using the genomics technology in animal models [22–25]. The marker genes identified in animal experiments are believed to be involved in the body weight loss of animals after WPV injection [25]. When considering an alternative assay, phenotypic changes in animals, such as body weight loss, cannot be assessed in cultured cells. On the contrary, marker genes linked to these bioactivities can be identified at the cultured-cell level. Biomarker genes can make it possible to link cellular data with biological reactions observed in animal phenotypes. We are currently working on demonstrating the usefulness of marker genes and their expression mechanisms. Most of the marker genes are involved in an immune response and are related to type 1 IFN signaling and innate immune responses [39]. According to these findings, it is possible that the usefulness of biomarker genes evaluated in animals can be extrapolated to cultured cells, if such cell lines as peripheral blood mononuclear cells, immune cells, and alveolar epithelial cell lines are employed in the assays. If an alternative (*in vitro* method) for the ATT and LTT is developed, it will be possible to secure the safety and quality of the current ATT and LTT by animal-free testing. This approach is expected to reduce the number of animals tested and to shorten the testing period.

8. Establishment of a new evaluation method for vaccine or adjuvant bioactivity based on biomarker gene function

Analysis by the genomics technology can be applied not only to the search for biomarkers but also to mechanistic analyses. Besides, it is possible to classify each biological reaction by hierarchical clustering analysis, according to microarray analysis results. Microarray analysis is the most information-rich assay; however, it is inefficient in terms of cost and labor. In the case of a clear-purpose test such as safety evaluation and quality control, it is expected that robust results will be obtained by using only selected highly important genes for evaluation. Therefore, if we consider the function of the genes identified as safety or quality evaluation markers for influenza vaccines, then the biological activity profile of the vaccine may be predicted. For example, genes such as *Irf7* are induced by type 1 IFN [55], genes such as *Psmb9* and *Tap2* are involved in antigen presentation [56], and *Csf1* participates in the activation of monocytes and macrophages [57]. Thus, expression levels of these genes could serve as indicators of the mode of action and help in the development of a biological activation assessment tool. These genes are thought to be involved in innate immunity, in which responses are observed at a relatively early time point after vaccination. Indeed, expression of these genes was assayed 16 h after vaccination. Therefore, long-term toxicity due to the vaccine (e.g., autoimmune and chronic inflammatory reactions) cannot be assessed. Safety evaluation by means of these biomarker genes is helpful for the development of adjuvant-containing vaccines. This is because most adjuvants are designed to activate the innate immune system. Adjuvants enhance innate immunity via cytokine production and activation of antigen-presenting cells; however, strong activation of innate immunity causes uncontrollable inflammatory reactions. This problem could lead to a fever, pain, and swelling, which appear as adverse reactions. Thus, adjuvants are required to have strong innate-immunity–activating effects, but at the same time, good safety. On the other hand, it is difficult to distinguish between the effectiveness and safety of vaccines. For example, interleukin (IL)-6 and type 1 IFN are important for the induction of adaptive immunity and are favorable for vaccine efficacy [58, 59]. Nevertheless, excess production of IL-6 or type 1 IFN causes a cytokine storm. Thus, safety can be evaluated with the same biological vector as that of effectiveness. In other words, if the factor of effectiveness becomes excessive, toxic effects may appear. We are currently working on establishing a safety assessment system based on the WPV as a toxicity indicator [60]. The WPV is an effective and excellent vaccine, but the frequency of adverse reactions is high, and currently, it is only rarely used, especially as a pre-pandemic vaccine. Therefore, we believe that the WPV can be a safety indicator. In other words, we think that there is a high probability that adjuvants and vaccines with innate-immunity–inducing activities that exceed the activity (toxicity) of WPVs will cause adverse reactions [60].

9. Future perspectives of safety evaluation of vaccines and adjuvants

According to the abovementioned concept, various evaluations of adjuvanted vaccines have been carried out. Furthermore, we have focused on the functions of biomarker genes. We have attempted to compile gene clusters based on the function of each gene. Such an assay is currently at the development stage, and further examination of the evaluation method and validation should be conducted in the future. Such an assay is considered applicable to the development of novel adjuvants.

For the development of low-molecular-weight synthetic drugs, a seed compound having a desired bioactivity is searched for by a screening system in compound libraries [61]. For promoting adjuvant development, to create as many prominent novel adjuvants as possible, finding seed compounds that are likely to become adjuvants is a crucial step in adjuvant development. Conventionally, to demonstrate whether a compound has adjuvant activities, animals are inoculated with one of the compounds, and the antibody titer and infection prevention rate are then assessed. This evaluation is not as efficient as the seed search and compound screening because the assessment process takes more than 1 month. In contrast, if we introduce an evaluation method involving a biomarker gene or genes, then prediction of safety and of the biological activity profile for compounds may be achieved in animals or cultured cells. Such an assessment may make it possible to search for effective adjuvant seeds that are safer than WPVs and more effective than the HAV.

10. Extrapolation of the safety evaluation results to humans according to biomarkers' gene function

Given that the evaluation of the quality and safety of vaccines assumes a reaction with humans, the evaluation result must reflect the human biological response. Generally, there are species differences in immunological responses between humans and rodents. Therefore, it is necessary to interpret the results carefully.

In case of safety evaluations based on genomic analyses, estimating the difference between experimental animals and humans with reference to the function of genes may be partially possible. For example, in the case of the WPV, leukopenic toxicity and body weight loss are observed in rodents, but these effects cannot be verified in humans. Nevertheless, at the gene level, if a gene is conserved among species, it is possible to estimate whether similar biological reactions can be observed between humans and animals. All our identified marker genes are homologous to their human counterparts, except for *Ifi47*. This observation suggests that some phenomena common to the tested animals and humans may be identified via the animal experiments by means of marker genes. To test this hypothesis and to develop an *in vitro* assay system, the use of human peripheral blood mononuclear cell-based or alveolar-epithelial-cell-based methods is necessary. Thus, extrapolation of the results of these evaluations to humans can be partially achieved by bridging the species differences with the marker genes.

11. Conclusions

It has been established that information that could not be obtained by conventional phenotypic analyses can be obtained by genomic analyses. Research conducted on the safety of vaccines and adjuvants using toxicogenomics has been less likely to be reported, and such data about chemically synthesized drugs have mostly been limited. Since the late 2000s, we have been trying to apply the genomics technology to the safety assessment of vaccines, and to demonstrate its sensitivity, ability to yield abundant toxicological and mechanistic information, the possibility of extrapolating its results to humans, and its potential for application to *in vitro* evaluation systems. In addition, we have shown that the newly developed evaluation system may be employed in analyses involving a biomarker gene(s) as an indicator, instead of the conventional quality control or safety test. It can also be assumed that these technologies can be utilized for adjuvant development, and it is expected that a wide range of genomics technologies will be applied in the future to the development of quality control and safety testing.

Acknowledgements

The research summarized in this review was supported by AMED, grant numbers JP17ak0101071 and JP17fk0108124.

Conflict of interest

The authors declare that they have no conflicts of interest.

Author details

Eita Sasaki, Takuo Mizukami* and Isao Hamaguchi

*Address all correspondence to: tmiz@nih.go.jp

Department of Safety Research on Blood and Biological Products, National Institute of Infectious Diseases, Musashimurayama, Tokyo, Japan

References

[1] Ulrich R, Friend SH. Toxicogenomics and drug discovery: Will new technologies help us produce better drugs? Nature Reviews. Drug Discovery. 2002;**1**:84-88

[2] Waters MD, Fostel JM. Toxicogenomics and systems toxicology: Aims and prospects. Nature Reviews. Genetics. 2004;**5**:936-948

[3] DeRisi J, Penland L, Brown PO, Bittner ML, Meltzer PS, Ray M, et al. Use of a cDNA microarray to analyse gene expression patterns in human cancer. Nature Genetics. 1996; **14**:457-460

[4] Schena M, Shalon D, Davis RW, Brown PO. Quantitative monitoring of gene expression patterns with a complementary DNA microarray. Science. 1995;**270**:467-470

[5] Wodicka L, Dong H, Mittmann M, Ho MH, Lockhart DJ. Genome-wide expression monitoring in Saccharomyces cerevisiae. Nature Biotechnology. 1997;**15**:1359-1367

[6] Nuwaysir EF, Bittner M, Trent J, Barrett JC, Afshari CA. Microarrays and toxicology: The advent of toxicogenomics. Molecular Carcinogenesis. 1999;**24**:153-159

[7] Boverhof DR, Zacharewski TR. Toxicogenomics in risk assessment: Applications and needs. Toxicological Sciences. 2006;**89**:352-360

[8] Ellinger-Ziegelbauer H, Gmuender H, Bandenburg A, Ahr HJ. Prediction of a carcinogenic potential of rat hepatocarcinogens using toxicogenomics analysis of short-term in vivo studies. Mutation Research. 2008;**637**:23-39

[9] Fielden MR, Brennan R, Gollub J. A gene expression biomarker provides early prediction and mechanistic assessment of hepatic tumor induction by nongenotoxic chemicals. Toxicological Sciences. 2007;**99**:90-100

[10] Gerecke DR, Chen M, Isukapalli SS, Gordon MK, Chang YC, Tong W, et al. Differential gene expression profiling of mouse skin after sulfur mustard exposure: Extended time response and inhibitor effect. Toxicology and Applied Pharmacology. 2009;**234**:156-165

[11] Huang J, Shi W, Zhang J, Chou JW, Paules RS, Gerrish K, et al. Genomic indicators in the blood predict drug-induced liver injury. The Pharmacogenomics Journal. 2010;**10**:267-277

[12] Low Y, Uehara T, Minowa Y, Yamada H, Ohno Y, Urushidani T, et al. Predicting drug-induced hepatotoxicity using QSAR and toxicogenomics approaches. Chemical Research in Toxicology. 2011;**24**:1251-1262

[13] Suter L, Haiker M, De Vera MC, Albertini S. Effect of two 5-HT6 receptor antagonists on the rat liver: A molecular approach. The Pharmacogenomics Journal. 2003;**3**:320-334

[14] Yang Y, Abel SJ, Ciurlionis R, Waring JF. Development of a toxicogenomics in vitro assay for the efficient characterization of compounds. Pharmacogenomics. 2006;**7**:177-186

[15] Zidek N, Hellmann J, Kramer PJ, Hewitt PG. Acute hepatotoxicity: A predictive model based on focused illumina microarrays. Toxicological Sciences. 2007;**99**:289-302

[16] McBurney RN, Hines WM, Von Tungeln LS, Schnackenberg LK, Beger RD, Moland CL, et al. The liver toxicity biomarker study: Phase I design and preliminary results. Toxicologic Pathology. 2009;**37**:52-64

[17] McBurney RN, Hines WM, Von Tungeln LS, Schnackenberg LK, Beger RD, Moland CL, et al. The liver toxicity biomarker study phase I: Markers for the effects of tolcapone or entacapone. Toxicologic Pathology. 2012;**40**:951-964

[18] Lühe A, Suter L, Ruepp S, Singer T, Weiser T, Albertini S. Toxicogenomics in the pharmaceutical industry: Hollow promises or real benefit? Mutation Research. 2005;**575**:102-115

[19] National Institute of Infectious Diseases, Minimum requirements for biological products, National Institute of Infectious Diseases, Japan; General Tests, 2006. p. 272-336. and p. 10-13. Influenza Vaccine

[20] Baylor NW, Midthun K. Regulation and testing of vaccines. In: Vaccines. Plotkin S, Orenstein W, Offit P, editors, 5th ed. Philadelphia: WB Saunders; 2008. p. 1611-1627

[21] Mizukami T, Masumi A, Momose H, Kuramitsu M, Takizawa K, Naito S, et al. An improved abnormal toxicity test by using reference vaccine-specific body weight curves and histopathological data for monitoring vaccine quality and safety in Japan. Biologicals. 2009;**37**:8-17

[22] Hamaguchi I, Imai J, Momose H, Kawamura M, Mizukami T, Kato H, et al. Two vaccine toxicity-related genes Agp and Hpx could prove useful for pertussis vaccine safety control. Vaccine. 2007;**30**:3355-3364

[23] Hamaguchi I, Imai J, Momose H, Kawamura M, Mizukami T, Naito S, et al. Application of quantitative gene expression analysis for pertussis vaccine safety control. Vaccine. 2008;**26**:4686-4696

[24] Momose H, Imai J, Hamaguchi I, Kawamura M, Mizukami T, Naito S, et al. Induction of indistinguishable gene expression patterns in rats by Vero cell-derived and mouse brain-derived Japanese encephalitis vaccines. Japanese Journal of Infectious Diseases. 2010;**63**:25-30

[25] Mizukami T, Imai J, Hamaguchi I, Kawamura M, Momose H, Naito S, et al. Application of DNA microarray technology to influenza A/Vietnam/1194/2004 (H5N1) vaccine safety evaluation. Vaccine. 2008;**26**:2270-2283

[26] Otto R. The state control of immunosera. In: Ehrlich P, editor. Work from the Royal Institute for Experimental Therapy in Frankfurt a. M. Vol. 2. Jena, Germany: Gustav Fischer; 1906

[27] Marxer A. Technology of Vaccines and Immunosera. Braunschweig, Germany: Friedr. Vieweg & Sohn; 1915

[28] Ortbals DW, Liebhaber H. Comparison of immunogenicity of a whole virion and a subunit influenza vaccine in adults. Journal of Clinical Microbiology. 1978;**8**:431-434

[29] al-Mazrou A, Scheifele DW, Soong T, Bjornson G. Comparison of adverse reactions to whole-virion and split-virion influenza vaccines in hospital personnel. CMAJ. 1991; **145**:213-218

[30] Xu W, Zheng M, Zhou F, Chen Z. Long-term immunogenicity of an inactivated split-virion 2009 pandemic influenza A H1N1 virus vaccine with or without aluminum adjuvant in mice. Clinical and Vaccine Immunology. 2015;**22**:327-335

[31] Momose H, Mizukami T, Kuramitsu M, Takizawa K, Masumi A, Araki K, et al. Establishment of a new quality control and vaccine safety test for influenza vaccines and adjuvants using gene expression profiling. PLoS One. 2015;**10**:e0124392

[32] Sasaki E, Momose H, Hiradate Y, Furuhata K, Takai M, Kamachi K, et al. Evaluation of marker gene expression as a potential predictive marker of leukopenic toxicity for inactivated influenza vaccines. Biologicals. 2017;**50**:100-108

[33] Mizukami T, Momose H, Kuramitsu M, Takizawa K, Araki K, Furuhata K, et al. System vaccinology for the evaluation of influenza vaccine safety by multiplex gene detection of novel biomarkers in a preclinical study and batch release test. PLoS One. 2014;**9**:e101835

[34] Cox RJ, Brokstad KA, Ogra P. Influenza virus: Immunity and vaccination strategies. Comparison of the immune response to inactivated and live, attenuated influenza vaccines. Scandinavian Journal of Immunology. 2004;**59**:1-15

[35] Soema PC, Kompier R, Amorij JP, Kersten GF. Current and next generation influenza vaccines: Formulation and production strategies. European Journal of Pharmaceutics and Biopharmaceutics. 2015;**94**:251-263

[36] Tamura SI, Asanuma H, Ito Y, Hirabayashi Y, Suzuki Y, Nagamine T, et al. Superior cross-protective effect of nasal vaccination to subcutaneous inoculation with influenza hemagglutinin vaccine. European Journal of Immunology. 1992;**22**:477-481

[37] Hasegawa H, Ichinohe T, Ainai A, Tamura S, Kurata T. Development of mucosal adjuvants for intranasal vaccine for H5N1 influenza viruses. Therapeutics and Clinical Risk Management. 2009;**5**:125-132

[38] Mutsch M, Zhou W, Rhodes P, Bopp M, Chen RT, Linder T, Spyr C, Steffen R. Use of the inactivated intranasal influenza vaccine and the risk of Bell's palsy in Switzerland. The New England Journal of Medicine. 2004;**350**:896-903

[39] Sasaki E, Kuramitsu M, Momose H, Kobiyama K, Aoshi T, Yamada H, et al. A novel vaccinological evaluation of intranasal vaccine and adjuvant safety for preclinical tests. Vaccine. 2017;**35**:821-830

[40] Robinson RA, DeVita VT, Levy HB, Baron S, Hubbard SP, Levine AS. A phase I-II trial of multiple-dose polyriboinosic-polyribocytidylic acid in patients with leukemia or solid tumors. Journal of the National Cancer Institute. 1976;**57**:599-602

[41] Cornell CJ Jr, Smith KA, Cornwell GG 3rd, Burke GP, McIntyre OR. Sytemic effects of intravenous polyriboinosinic-polyribocytidylic acid in man. Journal of the National Cancer Institute. 1976;**57**:1211-1216

[42] De Clercq E, Stewart WE, De Somer P. Interferon production linked to toxicity of polyriboinosinic acid-polyribocytidylic acid. Infection and Immunity 1972;**6**:344-347

[43] Gunzer M, Riemann H, Basoglu Y, Hillmer A, Weishaupt C, Balkow S, et al. Systemic administration of a TLR7 ligand leads to transient immune incompetence due to peripheral-blood leukocyte depletion. Blood. 2005;**106**:2424-2432

[44] Goldstein D, Hertzog P, Tomkinson E, Couldwell D, McCarville S, Parrish S, et al. Administration of imiquimod, an interferon inducer, in asymptomatic human immunodeficiency virus-infected persons to determine safety and biologic response modification. The Journal of Infectious Diseases. 1998;**178**:858-861

[45] Savage P, Horton V, Moore J, Owens M, Witt P, Gore ME. A phase I clinical trial of imiquimod, an oral interferon inducer, administered daily. British Journal of Cancer. 1996;**74**:1482-1486

[46] Tougan T, Aoshi T, Coban C, Katakai Y, Kai C, Yasutomi Y, et al. TLR9 adjuvants enhance immunogenicity and protective efficacy of the SE36/AHG malaria vaccine in nonhuman primate models. Human Vaccines & Immunotherapeutics. 2013;**9**:283-290

[47] Ato M, Takahashi Y, Fujii H, Hashimoto S, Kaji T, Itamura S, et al. Influenza A whole virion vaccine induces a rapid reduction of peripheral blood leukocytes via interferon-α-dependent apoptosis. Vaccine. 2013;**31**:2184-2190

[48] Garbe JHO, Ausborn S, Beggs C, Bopst M, Joos A, Kitashova AA, et al. Historical data analyses and scientific knowledge suggest complete removal of the abnormal toxicity test as a quality control test. Journal of Pharmaceutical Sciences. 2014;**103**:3349-3355

[49] Si-Tayeb K, Noto FK, Nagaoka M, Li J, Battle MA, Duris C, et al. Highly efficient generation of human hepatocyte-like cells from induced pluripotent stem cells. Hepatology. 2010;**51**:297-305

[50] Takayama K, Mizuguchi H. Generation of human pluripotent stem cell-derived hepatocyte-like cells for drug toxicity screening. Drug Metabolism and Pharmacokinetics. 2017;**32**:12-20

[51] Liang P, Lan F, Lee AS, Gong T, Sanchez-Freire V, Wang Y, et al. Drug screening using a library of human induced pluripotent stem cell-derived cardiomyocytes reveals disease-specific patterns of cardiotoxicity. Circulation. 2013;**127**:1677-1691

[52] Grimm FA, Iwata Y, Sirenko O, Bittner M, Rusyn I. High-content assay multiplexing for toxicity screening in induced pluripotent stem cell-derived cardiomyocytes and hepatocytes. Assay and Drug Development Technologies. 2015;**13**:529-546

[53] Novitsky TJ, Ryther S, Case MJ, Watson SW. Automated LAL testing of parenteral drugs in the Abbott MS-2. Journal of Pharmaceutical Science and Technology. 1982;**36**:11-16

[54] Cooper JF. Resolving LAL test interferences. Journal of Parenteral Science and Technology. 1990;**44**:13

[55] Ivashkiv LB, Donlin LT. Regulation of type I interferon responses. Nature Reviews. Immunology. 2014;**14**:36-49

[56] Groettrup M, Kirk CJ, Basler M. Proteasomes in immune cells: More than peptide producers? Nature Reviews. Immunology. 2010;**10**:73-78

[57] Stanley ER, Guilbert LJ, Tushinski RJ, Bartelmez SH. CSF-1 -a mononuclear phagocyte lineage-specific hemopoietic growth factor. Journal of Cellular Biochemistry. 1983;**21**: 151-159

[58] Tomljenovic L, Shaw CA. Mechanisms of aluminum adjuvant toxicity and autoimmunity in pediatric populations. Lupus. 2012;**21**:223-230

[59] Trinchieri G. Type I interferon: Friend or foe? The Journal of Experimental Medicine. 2010;**207**:2053-2063

[60] Sasaki E, Momose H, Hiradate Y, Furuhata K, Takai M, Asanuma H, et al. Modeling for influenza vaccines and adjuvants profile for safety prediction system using gene expression profiling and statistical tools. PLoS One. 2018;**13**:e0191896

[61] Szymański P, Markowicz M, Mikiciuk-Olasik E. Adaptation of high-throughput screening in drug discovery-toxicological screening tests. International Journal of Molecular Sciences. 2012;**13**:427-452

Section 7

Treatment of Influenza

Chapter 7

Therapeutic Approach for Seasonal Influenza and Pandemic

Yuji Takemoto

Additional information is available at the end of the chapter

http://dx.doi.org/10.5772/intechopen.76473

Abstract

Influenza infection is usually a self-limiting and suddenly life-threatening disease. Seasonal influenza causes severe clinical symptoms and almost subsides within 7 days in patients without severe illness, following no complications of pneumonia and encephalitis. Influenza A (H1N1) pdm09 brought the disaster including many deaths. We cannot make differential diagnosis between seasonal and pandemic influenza adequately in a pre-pandemic state. Seasonal influenza displaces suddenly pandemic, and we necessarily establish a standard treatment for influenza viral infection in routine work. If antiviral therapy would not be effective for patients with influenza viruses in an early period of illness, further investigations would be proceeded concerning three points: mutations of influenza viruses resistant to neuraminidase inhibitors (NAIs), concomitant diseases of patients, and a new pandemic virus. If the systemic procedure would be functioned, we are able to reduce individually burden of patients with severe clinical symptoms and leading complications and socially delay widespread of pandemic and plan for the streamline management of pandemic documents.

Keywords: antiviral therapy, seasonal epidemic, pandemic, streamline surveillance, the systemic procedure

1. Introduction

Influenza viruses spread seasonally and cause infection of the airway tract in humans following severe symptoms. Influenza viruses grow and multiply among in human, swine, and avian bodies. Influenza viruses escape human immunological protective system against influenza viruses by changing their epitope detected by human immune cells. Annual seasonal influenza epidemic often happened under no antiviral procedure by easy infection of influenza viruses.

Seasonal influenza viruses affect 10–20% of human population in epidemics each year [1] and worldwide, cause an estimated 3.5 million cases of severe illness and 250,000–500,000 death each year [2]. Although almost infected patients with seasonal influenza viruses recover from the disease in less than 2 weeks. On the other hand, some group of people containing young children, adults being elder than 65 years old and compromised hosts with severe illness had complications of influenza infection leading hospital admission [3]. Influenza viruses mutate and change the disease severity in host when transferring from avian to swine or from avian to human or from swine to human. A new mutant of influenza viruses is defined at the site of a mutation and called as influenza A (H5N1), A (H7N9), and A (H1N1) pdm09 each, causing severe affected people following many deaths [4]. Three influenza pandemics happened in the twentieth century: in 1918–1919, 1957, and 1968 and were called as Spanish flu, Asian flu, and Hong-Kong flu each and caused the severe disaster [4]. Especially Spanish flu brought estimated 20–50 million mortality [4]. We have the inability to predict and testify the appearance of dangerous influenza viruses to human health by the lack of rapid, affordable, highly sensitive, and specific diagnostic tests. The appearance of a new mutation of influenza viruses was noticed as unsuccessful treatment cases leading to life-threatening complications of influenza infection in the treatment of seasonal influenza [4]. The expansion of disaster by both the delayed use and little sharing of pre-pandemic information makes difficult in minimizing a widespread of a new mutant infection of influenza virus [4]. So it is necessary to establish a systemic procedure of diagnosis and treatment for patients with seasonal influenza and pandemic viruses in early phase of pandemic. In a first step of diagnosis of influenza virus infection, we can use rapid diagnostic kits for influenza A/B virus and we diagnose easily seasonal influenza infection in the outpatients. But rapid immune-chromatographic kits cannot show the mutation of influenza virus subtypes, we cannot make a differential diagnosis between seasonal and pandemic influenza virus by it [5]. A mutation of influenza virus subtypes is evaluated by reverse-transcriptase polymerase chain reaction (RT-PCR) and direct sequence of a recognition site of influenza virus subtypes [5]. This method is expensive and time-consuming. We cannot apply this method to all outpatients with influenza virus. On the course of clinical treatment, we need to discriminate patients with suspicious pandemic influenza virus from the other patients with seasonal influenza effectively and economically. We would discuss the feasibility and execution of this trial in the following chapters.

2. Prevention

It is not too enough to exaggerate that prevention is the most effective therapy for infectious disease. It is desirable to establish universal most effective vaccine against influenza virus. Vaccine effectiveness (VE) is influenced by viral subtype/lineage as well as the timing of vaccination (early or late epidemic in a season). VE of trivalent influenza vaccine (TIV) is assessed as from 20 to 50% in vaccine programs of several countries [6, 7]. The population rate of people was over 80% in the Korean national immunization program but VE remains low in the elderly adults [8]. They addressed the improvement of influenza vaccine including the adoption of quadrivalent influenza vaccine (QIV), adjuvanted influenza vaccine, and high-dose influenza vaccine. Recently, WHO has been recommending QIV in 2013 and QIV has been adopted in several countries. QIV is estimated cost-effective and cost saving to reduce the burden of outpatient visit for influenza but 1.62 hospitalizations and 0.078 deaths per 100,000 individuals were estimated in Japan [9]. VE is often influenced by the timing between vaccination and influenza epidemic. Early epidemic occurs seasonally before administration of vaccine against seasonal influenza infection in people and VE is low. A mismatch of influenza viral strains between vaccination and epidemic makes VE low. It is very difficult to overcome influenza infection only by vaccination because of current VE and variability of influenza virus. We need the adequate diagnosis and treatment systematically after the procedure of adequate vaccination.

3. Therapy for patients with influenza viruses

3.1. Antiviral therapy

Adoption of neuraminidase inhibitors (NAIs) for treating patients with influenza virus improves clinical incidences of outpatients leading hospitalization. Influenza infection is typical symptoms such as fever, headache, sore throat, cough, joints lasting, and sometimes diarrhea and nausea. On the first step of the treatment for influenza, concomitant use of antipyretic and mild analgesic drugs such as acetaminophen, are applied to the patients with influenza viruses as symptomatic treatment. It is very difficult to suppress widespread of influenza viruses without the isolation of patients within 1 or 2 weeks. On the next step of the treatment for influenza, amantadine and rimantadine were administered to patients with influenza A, and ribavirin was used to treat immunosuppressed patients with severe influenza conditions [10]. These are limited in operating only against influenza A viruses and adverse effect and resistance of virus to drugs lead to less use. On the use of these drugs, antiviral effectiveness for alleviation of severe symptoms of patients with seasonal influenza viruses was limited and not enough to suppress the widespread of those? On the third step of the treatment for influenza, NAIs are administered to the patients with influenza viruses. The NA protein is a homotetrameric glycoprotein with a stalk region and enzymatically active head. The NA active site cleaves sialic acid at the glycol-sialic bond on the host cell as well as in respiratory mucus, leading to spread of the virus [11–13]. NAIs act to inhibit the release of progeny viral particles from infected host cells and have more effectiveness and less adverse effects than amantadine and rimantadine when administered to patients with influenza viral infection [14]. Administration of NAIs to patients is recommended within 48 h from the onset of infection [14]. NAIs alleviate symptoms and shorten its duration bothered from typical symptoms of influenza, especially high fever and headache without using antipyretic agents. Four NAIs, namely oseltamivir, zanamivir, laninavir, and peramivir are available in various countries and three measures of administration, namely oral intake, inhalation, and infusion to vein are used [14]. Zanamivir was the first NAI to be developed and was licensed in 1999. Its feature is poor absorption and an inhaled agent and is available in an intravenous form for compassionate use [15]. Oseltamivir is a prodrug being developed on the basis of the structure of the active site of zanamivir and is activated in the liver [16]. Oseltamivir is administered orally and sometimes intravenously in the patients not being tolerable in oral dose [17]. Peramivir is administered only as an intravenous formulation and show low oral bioavailability [17]. It achieves very high concentration in the bloodstream and its half maximal inhibitory concentration (IC_{50}) for influenza viruses is lower than that of both oseltamivir and zanamivir [18]. Laninamivir is another inhaled prodrug which is activated in the respiratory tract. One inhalation of laninamivir is effective for patients with influenza virus because of long half-life and high concentration within tissue [17]. Now the adequate measure for administration of NAIs can be selected following as the patients' condition and ages. If patients are children and cannot intake NAIs orally or inhaler NAIs, intravenous infusion of peramivir would be recommended [19].

3.2. Necessity of monitoring body temperature in patients without antipyretic and analgesic drugs

Patients with seasonal influenza viruses almost have recovered from high-fever state within 1 or 2 days on the condition of no use of antipyretic drugs (**Figure 1**). So monitoring a patient's body temperature is useful to evaluate whether antiviral treatment is successful or not. We showed the typical monitor of successful treatment of NAIs in body temperature measured by

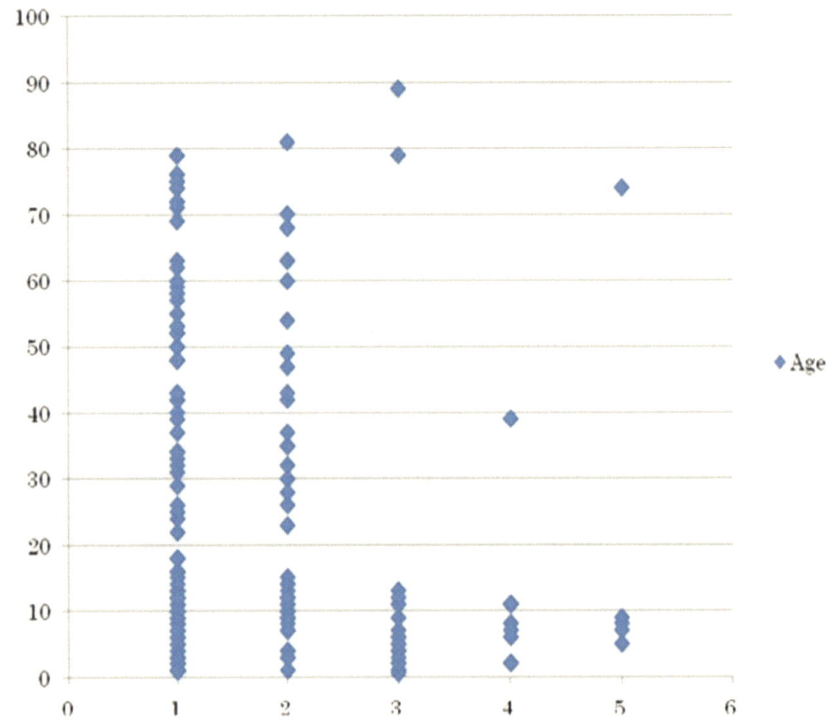

Figure 1. Correlation between age and amount of time required to alleviate fever. Almost cases with NAIs treatment have normal temperature within 3 days. This figure is cited from clinical effects of Oseltamivir, Zanamivir, Laninamivir, and Peramivir on seasonal influenza infection on outpatients in Japan during the winter of 2012–2013. Takemoto et al. [57].

the patient own (**Figure 2**). If treatment of NAIs fails to alleviate typical symptoms of patients with influenza viruses within 2–3 days, complications of influenza viral infection; influenza-associated pneumonia and encephalopathy would have to be investigated. The patient with influenza virus type A detected by a rapid test for influenza viruses had been annoyed over 4 days from onset of the disease on the condition of administration of zanamivir (**Figure 3**), and was diagnosed as influenza associated pneumonia by a close examination for further diseases (**Figure 4**). The antibiotic drugs were additionally administered to the patient (10-year-old girl) at the outpatient without antipyretic and analgesic drugs and pneumonia was treated successfully at home as the diagnosis of pneumonia categorized as mild severity and bacterial pneumonia following influenza viral infection. No new mutation of influenza virus A derived from this patient was detected. Hospitalization would be recommended for the severe pneumonia with any danger sign according to classification of pneumonia because pneumonia is the significant cause of death in the world [20, 21]. We had experienced one case of influenza-associated encephalopathy which had uncontrolled high fever and mild neuro-psychiatric disorder despite of administration of oseltamivir. We sent the 6-year-old boy to the hospital for diagnosis and treatment of influenza-associated encephalopathy and had good information of a full recovery without death or neurologic sequela. In all, 200–300 cases of influenza encephalopathy are reported as the result of 7% death, 17% survive with neurologic sequel, and 76% full recovery of patients in a year in Japan [22]. If high fever and other typical

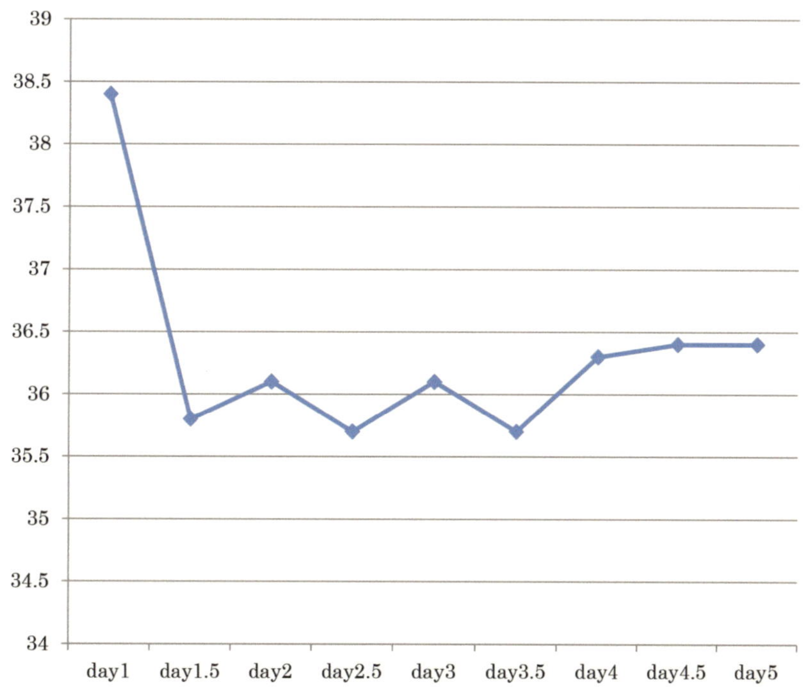

Figure 2. A pattern of body temperature of the patient with influenza virus A in the winter of 2017 is shown in a graph. The NAI is effective for alleviation of high fever and no relapse of fever in the effective clinical course of NAI treatment is shown. Patients with no complications and no resistant influenza viruses to NAIs show this pattern on the administration of NAIs.

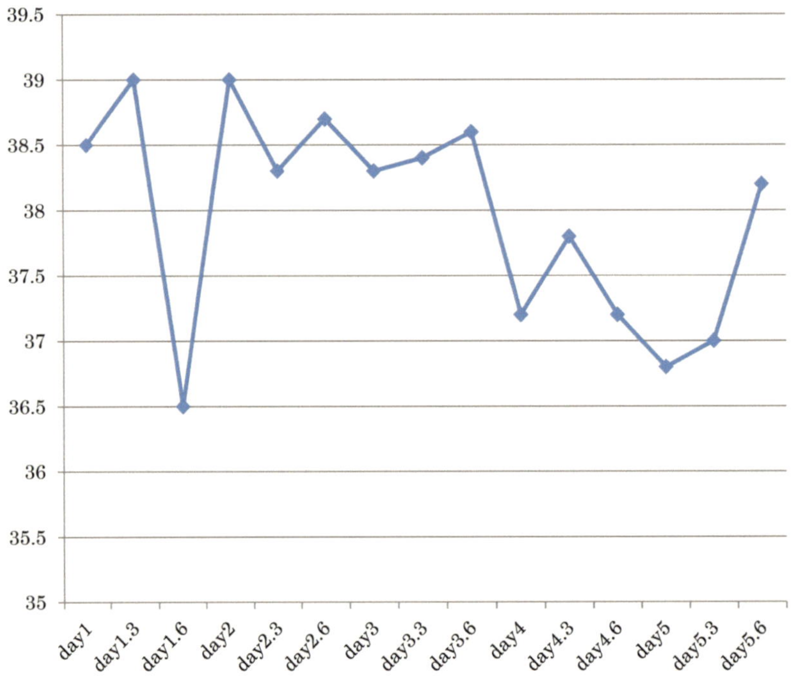

Figure 3. A pattern of body temperature of the patient with influenza virus A in the winter of 2017 is shown. High-grade fever is prolonged and relapsed over 3 days from the onset of influenza infection. Usually NAI treatment does not need the use of antipyretic agent for alleviation of high fever. Complications and/or viral mutations of resistant to NAIs cause the prolongation of high fever.

symptoms in patients with influenza viruses continue over 3–4 days under the administration of a NAI and no remarkable complications of influenza in patients, resistance of viruses to antiviral drugs or new mutations for pandemic should be investigated. It is very important to follow up patients in taking view of their body temperature from the beginning of NAI treatment and inform reconsultation with the doctors to patients on the condition of little amelioration from high fever of influenza infection within a few days.

3.3. NAIs were effective for influenza A (H1N1) pdm09

Pandemic of influenza A (H1N1) pdm09 was disseminated worldwide in 2009 –2010 and in many countries severe complications of its infection, hospitalization, and death from it were reported [23]. On the other hand, the incidence of such phenomenon was lower in a few countries than in the other countries. WHO overviewed pandemic 2009 on October in 2009 and defined the difficulty of comparison for evaluating the difference factors between countries due to the different age classes used to present data and the use of crude number of cases rather than rates [4]. The most burdened population of disease was occurred in younger age group as a striking difference between pandemic (H1N1) 2009 and seasonal epidemic [24]. This difference is hypothesized the population difference exposed to 1918–1919 epidemic like H1N1 influenza viruses between the elder generation over 65 years old and the younger

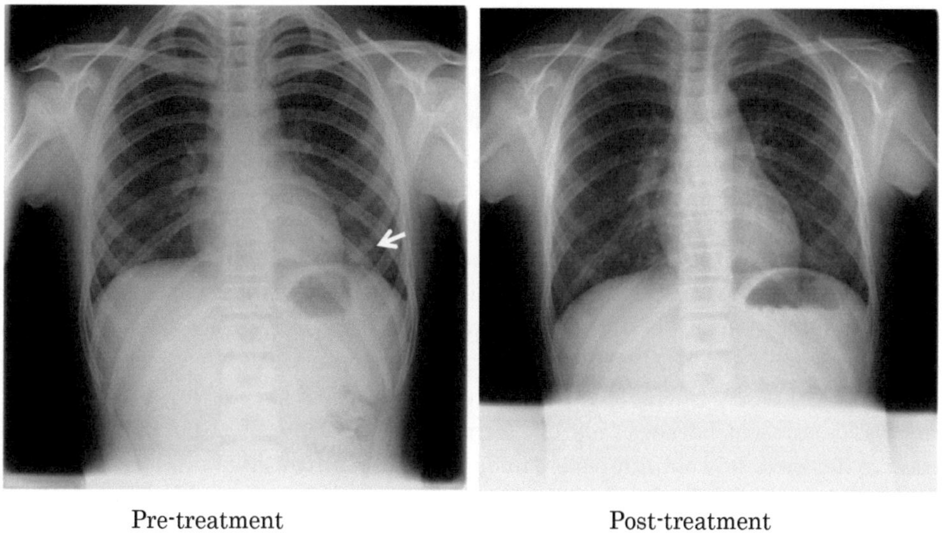

Figure 4. Chest X-ray films shows the influenza-associated pneumonia in the left lobe of the lung in the phase of pre- and post-treatment with antibiotics. Close examination for prolongation of high fever after treatment of NAI clarified the pneumonia in the patient with influenza virus infection in the early phase of pneumonia. A clinical treatment and follow up the patient with influenza virus with NAI and no antipyretic agents is useful for evaluation and findings of complications and viral mutations.

generation under 20. Compared with the rest of the population to develop severe disease, in countries of Americas and the Pacific, disproportionate affection by influenza A (H1N1) pdm 09 might be influenced by the prevalence of underlying medical conditions and limited access to medical care living conditions in addition to a social component and crowded living conditions [25]. Therefore, it is necessary to establish the medical conditions against viral infection and easy access to medical care in the worldwide for pandemic before administrating antiviral drugs. Adequate diagnosis of influenza infection and the early intervention with antiviral drugs (NAIs, etc.) to influenza viral infection among healthy little immunized population are desirable. On the other hand, effectiveness of NAI treatment is suggested for reducing mortality when given to hospitalized patients with influenza A (H1N1) pdm09 and the likelihood of requiring of hospital admission when given to population with confirmed or suspected influenza A (H1N1) pdm09 at high risk of hospitalization [26, 27]. NAI treatment following to rapid positive tests for influenza viruses might be effective for pandemic and reduce mortality rate of pandemic [27]. Additionally, influenza-like illness (ILI) in pandemic without laboratory confirmation among community patients with relatively severe influenza infection and patients with underlying comorbidities would be recommended to be treated by NAIs for reducing hospitalization and prevention of severity in early time (<48 h) after the onset of illness [26, 27].

3.4. Resistance to antiviral drug among influenza viruses

Influenza virus is a negative-sense RNA virus and contains eight gene segments that encode eleven proteins, including hemagglutinin (HA) and neuraminidase (NA) glycoprotein.

Influenza virus initiates the infection using HA to attach to sialic acid residues on the host cells and entries the host cells using M2 to initial receptor mediated endocytosis and releases progeny and propagate infection to other host cells using NA to cleave sialic acid residues on the host cells [28]. Each year influenza virus develops mutations within these genes leading antigenic drift and antigenic shift. Antigenic drift is represented by the little changed nature of virus and causes epidemics. Antigenic shift means change of major variant of virus and initiates a severe pandemic followed at intervals of a year or two by successive epidemics by antigenic drift [13]. Different from antigenic drift in transmission between interspecies by viruses, antigenic shift is the reassortment of gene segments between two different parental viruses within the same host [29]. The most recent pandemic; influenza A (H1N1) pdm09 was caused by a swine-origin H1N1 subtype, which originated from the sequential reassortment events between human H3N2, swine H1N1 subtype, and avian H1N2 subtypes of North America and Eurasian lineages [30]. Concerning to the nature of virus, many mutants of viruses are reported. It is not completely understood in mechanism to produce the resistance to antiviral drugs among influenza viruses. But many types of viruses being resistant to antiviral drugs are reported [31]. Adamantanes were the first approved class of antiviral drugs by binding M2 channel pore and blocking conductance either directly or allosterically. Consequently, adamantanes inhibits the virus RNA release and influenza virus replication [32]. Mutated amino acids (L26F, V27A, A30T/V, S31N, G34E, and L38F) in M2 membrane domain that line the channel pore (V27, A30, and G34) or are involved in the tetramer helix–helix packing (L26, S31, and L38), lead to increase in pore size with hydrophilicity of the channel or lead to narrow of the pore size with destabilization of helix–helix assembly. Consequently, influenza viruses reduced susceptibility to adamantanes [33]. In 1980 epidemics, the first detection of the resistance of influenza to adamantanes was reported [34]. The resistance of influenza viruses to adamantanes was rare with 1–2% frequently until 2000 [35] but the rate of resistance has dramatically risen to 27% since then [36]. From 2005 onward, the rate of the resistance to adamantanes started to increase almost exponentially to 90.6% of the H3N2 and the 15.2% of H1N1 global isolates [37]. Similar rates were confirmed in isolated viruses in the USA and the resistance conferring mutation was S31N in the 90–98% of isolated H1N1 and H3N2 subtypes [38]. Vast majority of adamantanes-resistant influenza virus subtypes (95%) contained the S31N mutation [39, 40]. Similar to M2, influenza virus has mutated several amino acids in or around neuraminidase active site to acquire the resistance to NAIs [41, 42]. Several in vitro and preclinical studies have found some mutations in neuraminidase; E119G/A/D/V, R292K, and H274Y [43]. Therefore, a global Neuraminidase Inhibitor Susceptibility Network (NISN) was established to monitor influenza virus to NAIs [44]. Unlike adamantanes resistance, which initially emerged and was predominant in H3N2 subtypes, NAI resistance first isolated and was spread in H1N1 subtypes [40, 45]. During the first 3 years of using NAI from 1999 to 2002, no resistance basically was detected [43, 44]. But from 2008 to April 2009 [before the emergence of influenza A (H1N1) pdm 09], over 99% influenza viruses of the H1N1 isolated were resistant to oseltamivir but were sensitive to zanamivir and none of the H3N2 isolates were resistant to oseltamivir in the report of the Centers for Disease Control and Prevention (CDC) in the USA [45]. Similarly in 2008–2009 season, more than 90% of the circulating H1N1 subtypes globally were oseltamivir resistant [46, 47]. H274Y mutant was predominantly circulating during 2008–2009 and rapid transmission of H274Y mutation in influenza (H1N1) pdm 09 has been detected in communities with little or no previous expose to oseltamivir [48, 49]. Fortunately, almost of the pandemic H1N1 global isolates collected between April 2009 and January 2010 were sensitive to NAIs, except an odd 0.7% and other few H1N1 isolated local cases [50–54]. The NAI sensitive 2009 pandemic H1N1 subtypes displaced the-pre-pandemic oseltamivir resistant H1N1 lineage and remains largely NAI sensitive and is predominantly circulating at present [54, 55]. Sequential investigation of influenza virus mutation following impairment of NAI treatment for seasonal epidemics is useful for early detection of pandemic. There is no rapid diagnostic test for the detection of mutation or strains available in clinical laboratories. Systemic reviews of influenza resistance to NAIs did not reveal any difference in time for alleviate symptoms between oseltamivir-resistant and oseltamivir-sensitive patients [56]. This conclusion is different from our data and this difference might be dependent on the different analysis between the monitor for fever isolated from symptoms and the monitor for all symptoms of patients including estimate difference [57]. On the course of NAI treatment, an alleviation time for fever is not over 2–3 days in the group of patients with seasonal influenza viruses susceptible to NAIs. Treatments for patients with influenza viruses resistant to NAIs are considered to switch to other NAI: oseltamivir to zanamivir or other NAIs or to combine two NAIs: oseltamivir and zanamivir or three antiviral drugs; oseltamivir, adamantanes, and ribavirin [58]. Evaluated by the outcome of influenza viral copy numbers at 48 h after treatment, dual therapy; zanamivir/oseltamivir is less effectiveness than oseltamivir monotherapy [59]. Triple combination antiviral drugs (TCAD) composed of oseltamivir, amantadine, and ribavirin impedes the selection of the influenza virus A in vitro and clinical trials have been completed for the treatment with immunocompromised hosts with influenza in the United States [60, 61]. For preparedness to emergence and widespread of influenza virus variants resistant to antiviral drugs, new antiviral agents targeting viral particles and mechanism of viral replication are desired. Polymerase inhibitors; T-705, VX-787, and S-033188 concerning to suppressing of replication, are undergoing phase 2/3 clinical trials and favipiravir (T-705) is approved for the treatment of pandemic in Japan [62] when NAIs are ineffective to pandemic and the government permit to use. In addition to new antiviral agents, pandemic vaccine is necessary for pandemic preparedness [5]. Genotypic and phenotypic assays are available in the surveillance laboratories. Genotypic assays are rapid and can be done without viral culture otherwise genetic resistance does not always correlate phenotypic resistance [63]. Phenotypic assays are able to the effect of both known and unknown resistant mutations coupled with genetic assays and provide susceptibilities to antiviral drugs [64]. World Health Organization (WHO) category based for NA inhibition assay is showed as follows: normal inhibition or susceptibility (S) (<10-fold increase in IC_{50} for influenza A, <5-fold increase for influenza B), reduced inhibition (RI) (between 10- and 100-fold increase for influenza A, between 5- and 50-fold increase for influenza B) and highly reduced inhibition (HRI) (>100-fold increase for influenza A, and >50-fold increase for influenza B [65]. All mutations were not definitely associated phenotypic resistance, but it is important to assess the relevance between clinical and phenotypic resistance to NAIs.

3.5. Strategy for treatment and survey

Nevertheless of clinical effectiveness and little adverse effects of NAI treatment for seasonal influenza infection, concerning about cost effectiveness of NAI treatment, conventional treatment was adopted for influenza infection in healthy populations without rapid tests for influenza viruses [66]. Effectiveness on NAIs in reducing mortality and hospitalization in patients with influenza A (H1N1) pdm09 was clarified [67]. Compared with no antiviral treatment, diagnostic testing and oseltamivir treatment when positive in children with seasonal influenza viruses is more effective and cost between $25,900 and $71,200 per quality-adjusted life year gained (QALY), depending on the prevalence of oseltamivir resistance in circulating viruses [68]. Oseltamivir treatment for influenza is less cost-effective than conventional treatment, considering the productivity loss by the analysis of the incremental cost-effective ratio (ICER) of oseltamivir in Japan [69]. Pandemic is consequent of unpredictable mutations of seasonal influenza and the only measure of the first information about pandemic is surveillance of an avian suspicious single death following cluster deaths or a report of clinical worsening cases of fevers unknown origin following severe complications in medication. The case of family cluster of a highly pathogenic avian influenza A (H5N1) virus might suggest for the hint of suppressing a widespread of viral infection to pandemic in Thailand in 2004 [70]. The index patient contacted with dying household chickens and 4 days later became ill and was presented to clinic with fever, cough, and a sore throat. The 11-year-old girl got worse in symptoms including fever and dyspnea within 5 days and was admitted for viral pneumonia and died in a day despite of intensive care. Her mother and aunt provided bedside care for her in the hospital for 18 h in 2 days and for 13 h in 1 day each. Her mother began to have high fever after 3 days of unprotected nursing care for her and was admitted to a hospital and died from pneumonia and progressive respiratory failure. Her aunt noted high fever, myalgia, and chills after 9 days of unprotected nursing care for her and was admitted to the distinct hospital. On the day of admission, the patient was suspected as pneumonia due to avian influenza and received treatment with oseltamivir and instituted full isolation precautions by an investigating team. Despite moderate dyspnea and hypoxia, she gradually ameliorated and was discharged a month later. First, a nasopharyngeal swab from the aunt was weakly positive for influenza nucleoprotein gene and no evidence of influenza infection in the laboratory data on tissue culture or egg inoculation. Specimens of lung obtained from the mother's body embalmed were positive for influenza A (H5N1) by RT-PCR at the Siriraj hospital laboratory in Thailand and at CDC in the United States. This study suggests that the systemic procedure of treatment for seasonal influenza is sequent to the systemic procedure of preparedness and response for the following pandemics and is desirable. The desirable systemic procedure for epidemic and pandemic is described as follow; [1] application of rapid tests for influenza virus in diagnosis, [2] early administration of NAIs within 48 h from a onset of influenza infection, [3] monitor for patients without antipyretic, [4] further investigation of complications and mutations of influenza viruses under late time of alleviation for fever, [5] adoption of other treatments for complications or hospitalization in the progression of illness, [6] check of family member or cluster by surveillance system if possible and consultation to public health center for the further investigation. After a new mutated influenza virus is confirmed, the isolation of the patients and the contacts are given antiviral prophylaxis and exposed persons are put under active surveillance and poultry in the surrounding area is culled under the control of government. This procedure would be helpful for treatment of seasonal influenza and the following pandemic. WHO recommend for development and application of measures to assess the severity of every influenza epidemic [5] and this procedure might be one of those? Addiction to measures to assess severity, strengthen surveillance technology is necessary to detect pandemic, too. There are four types of surveillance for seasonal influenza epidemic in Japan and one of those? is (Nursery) School Absenteeism Surveillance System ((N)SASSy) which enables real-time surveillance and informs its result to school officials including school lengths and teachers by websites [71]. This is one of tools for preparedness for epidemics: noticing each condition of the numbers of infected students with influenza virus, both inter-schools and inter-cities on the closed website and sharing real-time information for spread of epidemics around them. Open access to the website is available for spread of epidemics except personal information, names of schools, and so on. This surveillance system will be applied in pandemic as streamline surveillance in local. WHO suggests the Global Influenza Surveillance Network (GISN) and mobilize the Global Outbreak and Alert Response Network (GROAN) teams for information sharing [72]. WHO recommends a close relationship and partnership with International Health Regulations 2005 (IHR) to prevent and respond to acute public health risks worldwide [5]. Real-time surveillance and sharing of its information are useful in domestics and international.

4. Conclusions

Seasonal influenza virus mutates in transmission of interspecies and suddenly changes both highly lethal and transmissible from person to person. Prevention of influenza infection by universal vaccine is desirable but are undergoing in development. Confirmation for the emergence of pandemic influenza virus is only the detection of cluster infection with severe complications by the new mutated virus. Surveillance in local and global is the effective measure for it. We can add the procedure of clinical diagnosis and treatment for seasonal influenza infection to one of useful surveillance systems for pandemic. Adoption of NAIs and evaluation of clinical effectiveness monitoring body temperature is the first step of surveillance of clinical treatment. Assessment of NAI treatment insufficiency to influenza infection leads to the close examination for the factors of patients and viral mutations as the second step. In third step, antigenic drift and/or antigenic shift are examined on the condition of no patient's factors and information sharing for drug resistance and/or pandemic is necessary for administration of new antiviral drugs and combination therapy of antiviral drugs and/or the management against pandemic. It is difficult to predict when NAIs will not be ineffective to influenza infection due to viral resistance to those? New antiviral drugs for influenza virus are under development and they would change the treatment of influenza infection as NAIs changed it. If the new convenient and rapid diagnostic test for influenza viral infection of seasonal influenza virus and pandemic virus would be developed, it would be more useful than the clinical procedure. At present, the systemic procedure of treatment and taking measure for seasonal influenza infection in usual would lead to the preparedness and taking management against pandemic.

5. Future perspectives

Trial of antiviral therapy in influenza infection is progressed as in the treatment of hepatitis C viral infection and HIV infection, too. Now in influenza virus infection, the three mechanical points for viral inhibition in cells are applied and new drugs are developed. New NAIs and RNA polymerase inhibitor and the cap-dependent endonuclease inhibitor are in developed. Recently, baloxavir marboxil (trade name Xofluza) may be used within a few months in Japan and prevent viral replication by inhibiting the cap-dependent endonuclease activity of the viral polymerase instead of inhibition for viral release from host cells as NAIs act [73]. It inhibits influenza RNA viruses from hijacking the host mRNA transcription system to allow synthesis of viral RNA. Only oral one dose is effective for amelioration from symptoms of influenza viral infection with less adverse effects. New drugs and combinations for administration of antiviral drugs against influenza virus would be defined following to the appearance of new mutations concerning to drug resistance in the future. Seasonal influenza infection and pandemic would be under controlled by the application of antiviral drugs, vaccination, and surveillance.

Acknowledgements

Thanks to Teizabruo Asai, Itsuo Ikezoe, Takako Yano, Masahiro Ichikawa, Shogo Miyagawa, and Jun Matsumoto for supporting the clinical research for NAI treatment in 2012–2013 and membership in the Osaka Medical Association in Japan.

Conflict of interests

The author has no competing of interests to declare.

Author details

Yuji Takemoto

Address all correspondence to: y-t1@vesta.ocn.ne.jp

Kamijo Medical Office, Izumiotsu City, Osaka Prefecture, Japan

References

[1] World Health Organization. Health Topic, Influenza [Internet]. 2018. Available from: http://www.who.int/topics/influenza/en/ [Accessed: March 14, 2018]

[2] World Health Organization. Influenza, 25 January 2008 [Internet]. 2008. Available from: http://www.who.int/topics/influenza/en/.index.html [Accessed: March 14, 2018]

[3] Memoli MJ, Athota R, Reed S, et al. The natural history of influenza infection in the severely immunocompromised vs nonimmunocompromised hosts. Clinical Infectious Diseases. 2014;**58**(2):214-224. DOI: 10.1093/cid/cit725

[4] World Health Organization. Sixty Fourth World Health Assembly Provisional Agenda Item 13.2. 5 May 2011. Report of the Review Committee on the Functioning of the International Health Regulations in relation to Pandemic (H1N1) 2009 [Internet]. 2009. Available from: http://apps.who.int/gb/ebwha/pdf_files/WHA64/A64_10-en.pdf [Accessed: March 14, 2018]

[5] WHO Recommendations on the Use of Rapid Testing for Influenza Diagnosis. July 2005 [Internet]. 2005. Available from: http://www.who.int/influenza/resources/documents/RapidTestInfluenza_WebVersion.pdf [Accessed March 14, 2018]

[6] Andrew MK, Shinde V, Hatchette T, Ambrose A, Boivin G, Bowie W, et al., and on behalf of the Public Health Agency of Canada/Canadian Institutes of Health Research Influenza Research Network (PCIRN) Serious Outcomes Surveillance Network and the Toronto Invasive Bacterial Diseases Network (TIBDN). Influenza vaccine effectiveness against influenza-related hospitalization during a season with mixed outbreaks of four influenza viruses: A test-negative case-control study in adults in Canada. BMC Infectious Disease. BMC series-open inclusive and trusted. 2017;**17**:805. Published online 2017 Dec 29. DOI: 10.1186/s12879-017-2905-8

[7] Jackson ML, Phillips CH, Benoit J, Jackson LA, Gaglani M, Murthy K, HQ ML, Belongia EA, Malosh R, Zimmerman R, Flannery B. Burden of medically attended influenza infection and cases averted by vaccination United States, 2013/14 through 2015/16 influenza seasons. Vaccine. Jan 25, 2018;**36**(4):467-472:S0264-410X(17)31755-3. DOI: 10.1016/j.vaccine.2017.12.014

[8] Yun JW, Noh JY, Song JY, Chun C, Kim Y, Cheong HJ. The Korean Influenza National Immunization Program: History and present status. Infection & Chemotherapy. 2017; **49**(4):247-254. DOI: 10.3947/ic.2017.49.4.247

[9] Tsuzuki S, Schwehm M, Eichner M. Simulation studies to assess the long-term effects of Japan's change from trivalent to quadrivalent influenza vaccination. Vaccine. 2018;**36**(5): 624-630. DOI: 10.1016/j.vaccine.2017.12.058

[10] Hayden FG. Prevention and treatment of influenza in immunocompromised patients. The American Journal of Medicine. 1997;**102**(3, Supplement 1):55-60 ; discussion 75–76. DOI: 10.1016/S0002-9343(97)80013-7

[11] Nayak DP, Balogun RA, Yamada H, Zhou ZH, BS. Influenza virus morphogenesis and budding. Virus Research. 2009; Aug;**143**:147-161. DOI: 10.1016/j.virusres.2009.05.010

[12] Colman PM, Verghese JN, Laver WG. Structure of the catalytic and antigenic sites in influenza virus neuraminidase. Nature. 1983;**303**:41-44

[13] Hope-Simpson RE, Golubev DB. A new concept of the epidemic process of influenza A virus. Epidemiology and Infection. 1987;**99**:5-54

[14] Moscona A. Neuraminidase inhibitors for influenza. The New England Journal of Medicine. 2005;**353**:1363-1373. DOI: 10.1056/NEJMra050740

[15] Von Itzstein M, Wu WY, Kok GB, et al. Rational design of potent sialidase-based inhibitors of influenza virus replication. Nature. 1993;**363**:418-423. DOI: 10.1038/363418a0

[16] Kim CU, Lew W, Williams MA, et al. Influenza neuraminidase inhibitors possessing a novel hydrophobic interaction in the enzyme active site: Design, synthesis, and structural analysis of carbocyclic sialic acid analogues with potent anti-influenza activity. Journal of the American Chemical Society. 1997;**119**:681-690. DOI: 10.1021/ja963036t

[17] Samson M, Pizzorno A, Abed Y, Boivin G. Influenza virus resistance to neuraminidase Inhibitors. Antiviral Research. 2013;**98**(2):174-185. DOI: 10.1016/j.antiviral.2013.03.014

[18] Chairat K, Taming J, White NJ, et al. Pharmacokinetic properties of anti- influenza neuraminidase inhibitors. Journal of Clinical Pharmacology. 2013;**53**(2):119-139. DOI: 10.1177/0091270012440280

[19] Hikita T, Hikita H, Hikita F, Hikita N, Hikita S. Clinical effectiveness of peramivir in comparison with other neuraminidase inhibitors in pediatric influenza patients. International Journal of Pediatrics. 2012;**2012**:8341812. DOI: 10.1155/2012/834181

[20] Mackenzie G. The definition and classification of pneumonia. Pneumonia. 2016;**8**:14. [Internet]. Available from: https://doi.org/10.1186/s41479-016-0012-z [Accessed: March 14, 2018]

[21] WHO Library Cataloguing-in-Publication Data. Revised WHO Classification and Treatment of Pneumonia in Children at Health Facilities: Evidence Summaries 1. Pneumonia-Drug Therapy 2. Child 3. Health Facilities 4. Guideline I. World Health Organization. ISBN: 9789241507813 (NLM Classification: WA320) [Internet]. 2014. Available from: http://apps.who.int/iris/bitstream/10665/137319/1/9789241507813_eng.pdf [Accessed: March 14, 2018]

[22] Mizuguchi M. Influenza encephalopathy and related neuropsychiatric syndromes. Influenza and Other Respiratory Viruses;**7**(Suppl. 3):67-71. DOI: 10.1111/irv.12177. [Internet]. Available from: www.influenzajournal.com [Accessed: March 14, 2018]

[23] World Health Organization. Disease Outbreak News: Pandemic (H1N1)2009-UPDATE 112–6 Aug 2010 [Internet]. Available from: http://www.who.int/csr/don/2010 08 06/en/index/.html [Accessed: March 14, 2018]

[24] Bush R. Influenza forensics. In: Budolwe B et al., editors. Microbial Forensics. 2nd ed. London: Academic Press; 2011. pp. 109-135. [Internet]. Available from: http://www.sciencedirect.com/science/article/pii/B9780123820068000086 [Accessed: March 14, 2018]

[25] Writing Committee of the WHO Consultation on Clinical Aspects of Pandemic (H1N1) 2009 Influenza. Clinical aspects of pandemic 2009 influenza A (H1N1) virus infection. The New England Journal of Medicine. 2010;**362**:1078-1719. DOI: 10.1056/NEJMra1000494PMID.20445182. [Internet] 2010. Available from: http://www.nejm.org/doi/full/10.1056/NEJMra1000449 [Accessed: March 14, 2018]

[26] Venkatesan S, Myles PR, Bee JL, Muthuri SG, Masri MA, Andrew N, Bantar C, et al. Impact of outpatient neuraminidase inhibitor treatment in patients infected with influenza A (H1N1)pdm09 at high risk of hospitalization: An individual participant data metaanalysis. Clinical Infectious Diseases. 2017;**64**(10):1328-1334 . Published Online 2017 Feb 12. DOI: 10.1093/cid/cix127

[27] Louis JK, Yang S, Acosta M, Yen C, Samuel MC, Schechter R, Guevara H, Ueki TM. Treatment with neuraminidase inhibitors for critically ill patients with influenza A (H1N1) pdm09. Clinical Infectious Diseases. 2012;**55**(9):1198-1204

[28] Stouffer AL, Acharya R, Salom D, et al. Structural basis for the function and inhibition of an influenza virus proton channel. Nature. 2008;**451**(7178):596-599

[29] Worobey M, Han GZ, Rambaut A. Genesis and pathogenesis of the 1918 pandemic H1N1 influenza A virus. Proceedings of the National Academy of Sciences of the United States of America. 2014;**111**:8107-8112

[30] Neumann G, Noda T, Kawaoka Y. Emergence and pandemic potential of swine-origin H1N1 influenza virus. Nature. 2009;**459**:931-939

[31] Hussain M, Galvin HD, Haw TY, Nutsford AN, Husain M. Drug resistance in influenza A virus: The epidemiology and management infect. Drug Resistance. 2017;**10**:121-134. Published online 2017 Apr. 20. DOI: 10.2147/DR.S105473

[32] Schnell JR, Chou JJ. Structure and mechanism of the M2 proton channel of influenza A virus. Nature. 2008;**451**:591-595

[33] Cady SD, Schmidt-Rohr K, Wang J, Soto CS, Degrado WF, Hong M. Structure of the amantadine binding site of influenza M2 proton channels in lipid bilayers. Nature. 2010; **463**:689-692

[34] Heider H, Adamczyk B, Presber HW, Schroeder C, Feldblum R, Indulen MK. Occurrence of amantadine-and rimantadine-resistant influenza A virus strains during the 1980 epidemic. Acta Virologica. 1981;**25**:395-400

[35] Suzuki H, Saito R, Masuda H, Oshitani H, Sato M, Sato I. Emergence of amantadine-resistant influenza A viruses: Epidemiological study. Journal of Infection and Chemotherapy. 2003;**9**:195-200

[36] Bright RA, Medina MJ, Xu X, et al. Incidence of adamantane resistance among influenza A (H3N2) viruses isolated worldwide from 1994 to 2005: A cause for concern. Lancet. 2005; **366**:1175-1181

[37] Dong G, Peng C, Luo J, et al. Adamantane-resistant influenza A viruses in the world (1902–2013): Frequency and distribution of M2 gene mutations. PLoS One. 2015;**10**:e0119115

[38] Centers for Disease Control and Prevention (CDC). High levels of adamantane resistance among influenza A (H3N2) viruses and interim guidelines for use of antiviral agents—United States, 2005–06 influenza season. MMWR. Morbidity and Mortality Weekly

Report. 2006;**55**:44-46. [Internet]. 2006. Available from: https://www.cdc.gov/mmwr/preview/mmwrhtml/mm5502a7.htm [Accessed: March 14, 2018]

[39] Garcia V, Aris-Brosou S. Comparative dynamics and distribution of influenza drug resistance acquisition to protein M2 and neuraminidase inhibitors. Molecular Biology and Evolution. 2014;**31**:355-363

[40] Collins PJ, Haire LF, Lin YP, et al. Structural basis for oseltamivir resistance of influenza viruses. Vaccine. 2009;**27**:6317-6323

[41] Sheu TG, Deyde VM, Okomo-Adhiambo M, et al. Surveillance for neuraminidase inhibitor resistance among human influenza A and B viruses circulating worldwide from 2004 to 2008. Antimicrobial Agents and Chemotherapy. 2008;**52**:3284-3292

[42] Zambon M, Hayden FG. Global neuraminidase inhibitor susceptibility network. Position statement: Global neuraminidase inhibitor susceptibility network. Antiviral Research. 2001;**49**:147-156

[43] Monto AS, McKimm-Breschkin JL, Macken C, et al. Detection of influenza viruses resistant to neuraminidase inhibitors in global surveillance during the first 3 years of their use. Antimicrobial Agents and Chemotherapy. 2006;**50**:2395-2402

[44] Hurt AC, Barr IG, Hartel G, Hampson AW. Susceptibility of human influenza viruses from Australia and South East Asia to the neuraminidase inhibitors zanamivir and oseltamivir. Antiviral Research. 2004;**62**:37-45

[45] Dharan NJ, Gubareva LV, Meyer JJ, et al. Infections with oseltamivir-resistant influenza A (H1N1) virus in the United States. Journal of the American Medical Association. 2009;**301**: 1034-1041

[46] Baranovich T, Saito R, Suzuki Y, et al. Emergence of H274Y oseltamivir-resistant A(H1N1) influenza viruses in Japan during the 2008–2009 season. Journal of Clinical Virology. 2010; **47**:23-28

[47] Hurt AC, Ernest J, Deng YM, et al. Emergence and spread of oseltamivir-resistant A(H1N1) influenza viruses in Oceania, South East Asia and South Africa. Antiviral Research. 2009; **83**(1):90-93

[48] Takashita E, Kiso M, Fujisaki S, et al. Characterization of a large cluster of influenza A (H1N1)pdm09 viruses cross-resistant to oseltamivir and peramivir during the 2013–2014 influenza season in Japan. Antimicrobial Agents and Chemotherapy. 2015;**59**:2607-2617

[49] Hurt AC, Hardie K, Wilson NJ, et al. Characteristics of a widespread community cluster of H275Y oseltamivir-resistant A(H1N1)pdm09 influenza in Australia. The Journal of Infectious Diseases. 2012;**206**:148-157

[50] Gubareva LV, Trujillo AA, Okomo-Adhiambo M, et al. Comprehensive assessment of 2009 pandemic influenza A (H1N1) virus drug susceptibility in vitro. Antiviral Therapy. 2010; **15**:1151-1159

[51] Leung TW, Tai AL, Cheng PK, et al. Detection of an oseltamivir-resistant pandemic influenza A/H1N1 virus in Hong Kong. Journal of Clinical Virology. 2009;**46**(3):298-299

[52] Centers for Disease Control and Prevention (CDC). Oseltamivir-resistant 2009 pandemic influenza A (H1N1) virus infection in two summer campers receiving prophylaxis—North Carolina, 2009. MMWR. Morbidity and Mortality Weekly Report. 2009;**58**:969-972

[53] Centers for Disease Control and Prevention (CDC). Oseltamivir-resistant novel influenza A (H1N1) virus infection in two immunosuppressed patients—Seattle, Washington, 2009. MMWR. Morbidity and Mortality Weekly Report. 2009;**58**:893-896

[54] Dapat C, Kondo H, Dapat IC, et al. Neuraminidase inhibitor susceptibility profile of pandemic and seasonal influenza viruses during the 2009–2010 and 2010–2011 influenza seasons in Japan. Antiviral Research. 2013;**99**:261-269

[55] Hurt AC, Chotpitayasunondh T, Cox NJ, et al. Antiviral resistance during the 2009 influenza A H1N1 pandemic: Public health, laboratory, and clinical perspectives. The Lancet Infectious Diseases. 2012;**12**(3):240-248

[56] Thorlund K, Awad T, Boivin G, Thabane L. Systematic review of influenza resistance to the neuraminidase inhibitors. BMC Infectious Diseases. 2011;134. DOI: 10.1186/1471-2334-11-134

[57] Takemoto Y, Asai T, Ikeszoe I, Yano T, Ichikawa M, Miyagawa S, Matsumoto J. Clinical effects of oseltamivir, zabamivir, laninamivir and peramivir on seasonal influenza infection in outpatients in Japan during the winter 2012–2013. Chemotherapy. 2013;**59**:373-378

[58] Kamali A, Holodniy M. Influenza treatment and prophylaxis with neuraminidase inhibitors: A review. Infection and Drug Resistance. 2013;**6**:187-198. DOI: 10.2147/IDR.S36601

[59] Dual X, van der Werf S, Blanchon T, et al. Efficacy of oseltamivir-zanamivir combination compared to each monotherapy for seasonal influenza: A randamaized placebo-controlled trial. PLoS Medicine. 2010;**7**(11):e100032

[60] Hoops JD Driebe EM, Kelley E, et al. Triple combination antiviral drug (TACD) composed of amantadine, oseltamivir, and ribavirin impedes the selection of drug-resistant influenza A virus. PLoS One. 2011;**6**(12):E29778

[61] Fred Hutchinson Cancer Research Center. TACD vs Monotherapy for Influenza A in Immunocompromised Patients. Available from: http://clinicaltrials.gov/show/NCT00867139. NLMidentifier:NCT00867139

[62] Fukuda Y, Takahashi K, Fukuda Y, Kuno M, Kamiyama T, Kozai K, Nomura N, Egawa H, Minami S, Watanabe Y, Narita H, Shiraki K. In vitro and in vivo activities of anti-influenza virus compound T-705. Antimicrobial Agents and Chemotherapy. 2002:977-981

[63] Okumo-Adhiambo M, Sheu TG, Gubareva LV. Assay for monitoring susceptibility of influenza viruses to neuraminidase inhibitors. Influenza and Other Respiratory Viruses. 2013;**7**:44-49

[64] Gubareva LV, Webster RG, Hayden FG. Detection of influenza virus resistance to neuraminidase inhibitors by the enzyme inhibition assay. Antiviral Research. 2002;**53**:47-61

[65] World Health Organization [Internet]. Available from: http://www.who.int/influenza/gisrs_laboratory/antiviral_susceptibility/nai_overview/en/ [Accessed: March 14, 2018]

[66] Allan J, Alexander W, Sutton J, Cooper NJ, Turner DA, Abraham KR, Brennan A, Nicolson KG. Cost-effectiveness and value of information analyses of neuraminidase inhibitors for the treatment of influenza. Value in Health. 2008;**11**(2):160-171. DOI: 10.1111/j.1524-4733.2007.00241.x

[67] Muthuri SG, Venkatesan S, Myles PR, Bee L, et al. Effectiveness of neuraminidase inhibitors in reducing mortality in patients admitted to hospital with influenza A H1N1pdm09 virus infection: A meta-analysis of individual participant data. The Lancet Respiratory Medicine. 2014;**2**:395-404. DOI: 10.1016/S2213-2600(14)70041-4

[68] Lavelle TA, Uyeki TM, Prosser LA. Cost effectiveness of oseltamivir treatment for children with uncomplicated seasonal influenza. The Journal of Pediatrics. 2012;**160**(1):67-73

[69] Nagase H, Moriwaki K, Kamae M, Yanagisawa S, Kamae I. Cost-effectiveness analysis of oseltamivir for influenza treatment considering the virus emerging resistant to the drug in Japan. Value in Health. 2009;**12**(Supplements 3):62-65

[70] Ungchusak K, Auewarakul P, Dowell SF, Kitphati R, Auwanit W, Puthavathana P, Uiprasertkul M, Boonnak K, Pittayawonganon C, Cox NJ, Zaki SR, Thawatsupha P, Chittaganpitch M, Khontong R, Simmerman JM, Chunsutthiwat S. Probable person-to-person transmission of avian influenza A (H5N1). The New England Journal of Medicine. 2005;**352**(4):333-340. DOI: 10.1056/NEMJMoa044021

[71] Shimatani N, Sugishita Y, Sugawara T, Nakamura Y, Ohkusa Y, Yamagishi T, et al. Enhanced surveillance for the sports festival in Tokyo 2013: Preparation for the Tokyo 2020 Olympic and Paralympic games. Japanese Journal of Infectious Diseases. 2015;**68**:288-295

[72] Heymann D, Kindhausser M, Rodier G. Coordinating the global response. In: Sars: How a Global Epidemic was Stopped. Manila: WHO Regional Office for the Western Pacific; 2006. pp. 49-55. DOI: 10.2471/BLT.07.032763

[73] A Study of S-033188 (Baloxavir Marboxil) Compared with Placebo or Oseltamivir in Otherwise Healthy Patients with Influenza (Capstone 1) [Internet]. 2018. Available from: https://clinicaltrials.gov/ct2/show/NCT02954354 [Accessed: March 14, 2018]